YOGA FOR BODY, BREATH, AND MIND

YOGA FOR BODY, BREATH, AND MIND

A Guide to Personal Reintegration

A.G. Mohan

edited by Kathleen Miller

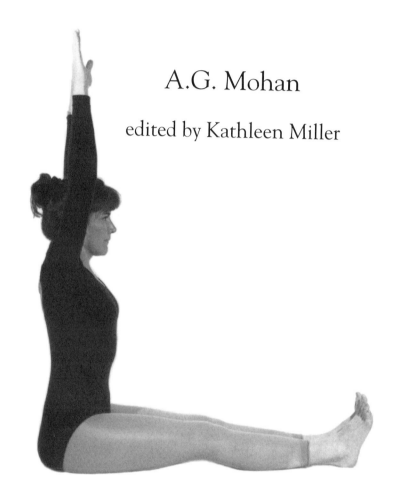

Rudra Press
Portland, Oregon
and
International Association of Yoga Therapists
Los Angeles, California

Rudra Press
P.O. Box 13390
Portland, OR 97213
Telephone: 503-235-0175
Telefax: 503-235-0909

International Association of Yoga Therapists
4150 Tivoli Avenue
Los Angeles, CA 90066

Cover Design: Bill Stanton
Text Design: Susan Cobb and Lubosh Cech
Illustrations: Hannah Bonner and Laura Santi
Photographs: Patrick Riordan

Manufactured in the United States of America.

This book is not intended to replace medical advice. The author and publisher urge you to verify the appropriateness of any procedure or exercise with your qualified health care professional. The author and publisher disclaim any liability or loss, personal or otherwise, resulting from the procedures and information in this book.

Library of Congress Cataloging-in-Publication Data

Mohan, A.G. (Angarai Ganesha), 1945 -
     Yoga for body, breath, and mind : a guide to personal
reintegration/A.G. Mohan; edited by Kathleen Miller.
        p.   cm.
     Includes index.
     ISBN 0-915801-51-5 : $16.95 USA
     1. Yoga, Hatha.   I. Miller, Kathleen.   II. Title
RA781.7.M64   1992
613.7'046--dc20   92-32175
                                                                CIP

98 99 00 01   10 9 8 7

Dedicated to
Samkhya Yoga Sikhamani, Vedanta Vageesa, Veda Kesari,
Nyayacharya Mimamsa Tirtha, Mimamsa Ratna, Yogacharya
Shri T. Krishnamacharya

Please note: We have romanized the Sanskrit phonetically in this text. Therefore ś = sh (for example śavāsana = shavasana), and c = ch (for example cakra = chakra).

CONTENTS

EDITORS' INTRODUCTION

In the modern West, the concept of personal reintegration stands in direct contrast to what many of us experience as a response to the pressures of our daily lives — most notably, the experience and symptoms of stress. This state of chronic disturbance seems to have become nearly endemic.

On the more superficial levels, the experience of stress expresses itself through such symptoms as nervous hand tapping, an upset or tight stomach, or difficulty in breathing smoothly and naturally. On a deeper level, such tension affects all levels of the person. It can have effects on the immune system and on one's general state of health and well-being in ways that may take years to develop, and which can ultimately become life-threatening.

Usually we assume that the causes of stress are external ones. This happened, or that happened, creating the stressful situation. Yet, according to yogic thought, the basic cause of the problem lies in the mind. If the mind perceives something as an obstacle or a threat, the body reacts with a fight or flight response although, in most cases, our social conditioning prevents us from actually doing the one or the other. Instead, adrenalin may be pumped into the system, digestion may be impaired, the muscles may tighten, and so on.

Ironically, however, what we generally perceive to be the external causes of our distress reduces, in fact, to a single, internal cause: our mind's reaction to an event or situation. The actual event itself cannot be directly linked to the specific bodily effects. Think, for example, of how on a bad day, it takes very little to provoke a strong reaction, whereas on other days the same situation may seem no more significant than tripping over your shoelace. What makes the difference is our state of mind. When our perception is clear, we are able to see things as they really are and to deal with them in a balanced, steady, flexible way. When we lose this clarity and our perceptions become clouded, we experience stress and react accordingly.

In order to bring ourselves back into an integrated state, the simplest way is to deal with the basic cause of our distress — the root of the problem. Instead of trying to tackle things on the level of various specific problems and dilemmas, yoga aims to remove the obstacles to clear perception, thereby achieving clarity of mind. Yoga is the means for removing these obstacles, or what are referred to in the tradition as "impurities" (*kleshas*). In fact, a practice that does not accomplish this cannot truly be called yoga.

Yoga addresses the immutable link between the body, the breath, and the mind, recognizing that any conscious attempt to modify one of these factors can be used as an agent for comprehensive change in the entire system. Therefore, for example, the first step in the path toward accurate perception — as well as toward freedom from suffering — is to learn how to keep the body and breath in their optimal state of balance and health. The practice of postures is the vehicle for that process. However, in the West the practice of postures (*asana*) and yoga have become synonymous.

The ideal forms of asana — these physical postures in the practice of yoga — come from ancient texts that reflect a manner of teaching quite different from what we frequently encounter in the modern West. Here in the West, for the most part, adult students have only some set of ideal poses in a book with which to work. Either that, or they see poses performed by an instructor in a video or in a group class, which they must then try to imitate. The essence of the practice of postures — to bring about a state of reintegration — is lost.

In ancient days in India, it was customary for a boy of eight years of age to begin instruction with a master, with whom he lived. This teacher became deeply involved with all areas of the boy's life and, therefore, knew him intimately. The actual yoga practice consisting of postures, breathing, and meditation was taught to the boy individually, based on the teacher's knowledge about him. It therefore incorporated practices that were specifically appropriate for him, and which were selected to promote his growth in a fully integrated way.

These adaptations to the boy's individual capacities and needs also had the advantage of working with a young body and a fresh mind, all of which made learning yoga quite a different experience from what many people have experienced here in the West. What gets lost here is not only the relationship with the teacher, but also the highly refined process of adapting the practice to fit the student, with the aim of bringing about a state of full, personal reintegration.

Indeed, the greater aim of yoga practice is to bring about such a state of personal reintegration. This kind of practice must grow out of the specific conditions and circumstances of the individual. The understanding of how to develop a yoga practice that takes into consideration the needs of the individual student is one of the important features that distinguishes the yoga taught by A.G. Mohan.

Based on his studies with his own teacher, Shri T. Krishnamacharya, one of the great exponents of yoga in the modern era, Mohan — together with his wife Indra — presents here some of the tools and understanding necessary to putting together a yoga practice designed to bring about the state of personal reintegration. Indra herself received a post-graduate diploma from Shri Krishnamacharya and, out of her own dedication to his teaching, has worked for more than a decade as a yoga teacher. She is deeply versed not only in the art of teaching yoga, but in the life that *is* yoga. She brings this depth of insight and experience to complement the work of Mohan.

This book intends to convey some of what Mohan and Indra have found to be most precious in the transmission from teacher to student: the understanding of the practice of yoga as a profound process of personal growth and wholeness. It is our great pleasure to share their work with you.

The Editors

FOREWORD
by Shri T. Krishnamacharya

श्री हयग्रीवाय नमः

हरिः ओम् । एका विज्ञप्तिः अत्यन्त सन्तोष पूर्विका ।

वरीवर्ति चरीकर्ति भरीभर्ति च लीलया ।
सञ्जरीकर्ति यो देवः वासुदेवः स पातु वः ॥

प्रिय मित्राणि ! प्रियबान्धवाः ! विद्वत् गणाश्च ! श्रद्धया इदं वाक्यपुञ्जं शृण्वन्ति इति दृढं विश्वसिमि । शृण्वतां अपि आश्चर्यावहं वृत्तम् यत् अत्यल्पेभ्यः दिनेभ्यः मत् छात्रः ब्रह्मश्री मोहन नामकः यः प्राक् शिल्पकलायां निपुणो भूत्वा, उत्तम वेतनं प्राप्य, गृहस्थो भूत्वा, भगवदनुप्रहात् सत्सन्तानवान् कतिपयकालं परिहाप्य, न जाने कारणं, अत्रैव मद्रास् नगरे प्रचलन्त्यां योगमन्दिरनामिकायां शालायां, रहस्यं प्रात्यक्षिकप्रदर्शनेन सः योगासनादि, शिक्षन् सन् न केवलं स्वयं, अन्यान् पातञ्जलमतरीत्या स्वाभ्यस्त योगविद्यां शिक्षयन्, योगशालां वृद्धिं नीतवान् इति सार्वजनीनम् ।

विशेषतस्तु अयं भारद्वाज गोत्रिकः वैदिक वंशसन्तानीयः । अस्य पिता श्रीमान् गणेश नामा इत्यन्यदेतत् । अनेन मन्निकट एव पातञ्जल योगारव्य अभ्यासः कृतः । न केवलं तावन्मात्रमेव, तादात्विकसमयप्रभृति अद्यावत् योगाभ्यासस्य ये योगाः, यानि यानि उपयोग करणानि, तानि सर्वाणि अभ्यस्यन्; कथंचित् मत्पुत्रेण वेङ्कट देशिकाचार्य नाम्ना सतीर्थ्यतां अवाप । एकाधिक संख्याविद्यार्थिनः एकस्मिन् गुरौ एक विषयमधिकृत्य अधीत्य, साङ्गवेद अध्ययनानन्तरं, गुरुकुलात् समावर्तन्ते ते एकगुरवः सतीर्थ्याश्च । तेषां अनूचानाः इति प्रसिद्धिः । "अनूचानः प्रवचने साङ्गेऽधीती गुरोस्तु यः । लब्धानुज्ञः समावृत्तः" इति अमरसिंहः । इदानीं मत्पुत्र ब्रह्मश्री वेङ्कटदेशिक, मोहनशर्मणोः यथाकथंचित् एवंरूपं अनूचानत्वं सतीर्थ्यत्वम् । तत्रैव अमरसिंहः । "सतीर्थ्याः तु एकगुरवः" इति जगाद । तेन अपात्रे शास्त्रस्य व्ययः न कृतः इति निश्चीयते ।

एको वा द्वौ वा त्रयोवा विद्यार्थिनः एकस्मिन् गुरौ एक विषयकं भिन्न भिन्न विषयकं वा शास्त्राध्ययनं कुर्वन्तु कामम् । अयं तु मोहन नामकः मन्निकट एव पातञ्जल योग शास्त्रं अधीत्य, प्रत्यक्षेण अभ्यस्य, कस्य कीदृशं आसनं प्राणायामं च योग्यं? कस्य कीदृशं आसनं प्राणायामं च अयोग्यं? इति विषयं ज्ञात्वा अध्यापयितुं समर्थः । आसनप्राणायामानां च अवान्तरभेदाश्च ये ये शास्त्रेषु इतरेषु उक्ताः तानि सर्वाणि अध्यापयितुं शक्नोति । तानि सर्वाणि मूलतः जानाति । एवं अनेन मोहनेन सांख्यतत्वटीका समग्रा अधीता । आयुर्वेद शास्त्रे – निदान स्थान, चिकित्सा स्थान, विमान स्थान, गर्भस्थान – विषयेषु मुख्यांशः अधीताः । भगवत्पूजादि विषये समाश्रयणमन्तरा प्रपदनमन्तरा संग्रहभागाः, तत् संप्रदायानुगुणाः अधीताः । कर्म काण्डविषये- पुण्याहवाचन, औपासन, समिदाधान – इत्यादीनि संग्रहतः प्रात्यक्षिकप्रदर्शनरूपतया च अधीतानि । मन्त्र भागविषये – नारायण अष्टाक्षर, वासुदेव द्वादशाक्षर इत्यादि महामन्त्रस्य मूल, अनुष्टुप्, षडक्षर रूपाः रहस्य भागाः, मालामन्त्रभागाश्च अधीताः । सर्व वेदान्तेषु गीता अधीता, उपनिषदः कतिपयाः अधीताः। ब्रह्म सूत्राणि अध्ययनार्थं आरब्धानि । प्रथम पादः प्रचलति । संप्रदाय मन्त्र भागे आधुनिक पूर्ववयस्कानां न तावती श्रद्धा तत्र । अयं तु इदानीं अपि अधीते । मोहनस्य मङ्गलमस्तु ।

सर्व शम् ।

FOREWORD*

Hayagrivaya Namah, Hari Om
Salutations to Lord Hayagriva

With great happiness I send forth this message. Let Lord Vasudeva, who is all pervasive and omnipresent, who is responsible for all actions, who supports the whole world, and who performs all these these things playfully, protect us all.

Friends, dear relatives, and learned persons, I sincerely wish that all of you may earnestly listen to me. By good fortune, my student Mohan, who was an engineer by profession and earning a good salary at this work, who is married and blessed with good children, has learned all the *yogashastras* (the science of yoga) in a practical manner, in a short period of time. It is known to all that he has also helped in the development of the yoga Mandiram at Madras, as well as spreading the message of yoga in the order of Patanjali, and practicing himself.

He was born in the Bharadawaja gotra, in a pious Vedic family. His father's name is Ganesha. All these things apart, he directly learned all of the different aspects of yoga and its practical usage from me, and became a colleague — *sathirthya* — of my son, Venkata Desikachar.

If more than one student studies the same subject, such as the *Vedas* and their *angas* (auxiliary subjects), under the same *Guru*, or teacher, these students are called sathirthyas. They are also called *Anucanah*. Amarasimha (author of *Amarakosa*, the sanskrit lexicon) says, "Anucana is one who has learnt the Vedas and its angas, one who has the ability to teach and express himself, who has taken to *Grahasthashrama* (householdership) after completion of studies with his Guru."

Now my son Venkata Desikachar and Mohanasarma, who are jointly studying under me, have attained this status of sathirthyas. Sathirthya means "studied under one Guru," says Amarasimha. This gives me the satisfaction

*translated from sanskrit

that I have not taught the shastras (the sacred treatise) to an undeserving person. Let one, two, or many students learn from one teacher about a particular subject, or varied subjects or shastras.

But what is special here is that Mohan has studied the *Patanjali Yoga Sutras* and its practical application entirely from me. He is competent to teach *asana* and *pranayama* suitable to each individual. He is also competent to teach the asana and pranayama portions of other shastras which he has studied thoroughly. He has studied the *Samkhya* philosophy in depth. In Ayurveda he has studied the important portions of *Nidana sthanam* (diagnosis), *Cikitsa sthanam* (treatment), *Vimana sthanam* (causes of disease), and *Garbha sthanam* (constitution of body). In *Bhagavad Puja* (prayer practices) excluding *Samasrayanam*, *Pravadanam* and *Prapatti*, he has learnt the texts comprehensively, in keeping with his tradition.

In rituals (*Karmakanda*) he has learnt *Punyakavacanam*, *Aupasanam*, and *Samitadanam* in a brief but practical manner. As far as the *Mantra Shastras* (the science of mantras) are concerned he has learnt the *Mula*, *Anushtup*, and so on, of the *Mahamantras* like the *Narayana Ashtakshari*, *Vasudeva Dvadashakshari*, apart from the secret portions of *Shadakshara* and *Malamantra*. Among the Vedanta texts the *Bhagavad Gita* has been completed by him. He has also studied some of the important *Upanishads*. He has just begun to study the *Brahma Sutra*. The first *padam* (section) of the first chapter is going on.

Nowadays most people who belong to the younger generation are not interested in the study of the vedas and mantras. But Mohan has great interest in this and continues to study. Let everything be well with Mohan. Let there be peace and prosperity everywhere.

Shri T. Krishnamacharya
December 22, 1988

AUTHOR'S INTRODUCTION

In November of 1988, I found myself reflecting during an unusual centenary celebration. It was the one hundredth birthday of my *Acharya*, Shri Krishnamacharya. Still hale and hearty, he had lived a full and satisfying hundred years. He was a true yogi. How often does one experience the centenary celebration of a living legend?

Shri Krishnamacharya devoted a considerable portion of his time between his eighty-third and hundredth year to tutoring me in the study of yoga. One of his constant refrains was that yoga must be adapted to the individual, and that it should lead to reintegration. This was at the heart of everything he taught me.

For some time, I deliberated as to how I could pay my debt of gratitude to this great master. From ancient times, the way to do so was to spread the essence of the teaching. I therefore decided that I should do the same.

I approached my teacher, expressing my wish to write a book, and asked him if he would bless me in my endeavor with an introduction. Instead, he dictated an introduction not about the book but about my studies with him, and then blessed me in my endeavor. This is presented as the foreword to this book.

With this blessing, I started to write the book itself. This endeavor has been brought to completion through seminars I conducted for the International Association of Yoga Therapists (IAYT), and at the Nityananda Institute in Cambridge, Massachusetts, in the United States.

I deeply thank Shri T.K.V. Desikachar, who has taught me a great deal and who has extended me great support during the last two decades of my career as a teacher of yoga. My thanks are also due to Swami Chetanananda,

Abbot of the Nityananda Institute, for his support, his inspiration, and for the actual publication of the book.

Even more than thanks go to my wife, Indra, and to my friend S.V. Subramanyam, who have been involved in every aspect of this book, including the original formulation, the writing, and the editing. They have my profound gratitude.

I would also like to thank the many others who have helped me in this endeavor including Sharon Ward of the Nityananda Institute, Larry Payne of the International Association of Yoga Therapists, and Claude Cooke for his generous support. The efforts of Kathleen Miller, Rachel Gaffney, Linda Barnes, Nanette Redmond, Robert Flickinger and Jeffrey S. Miller brought the manuscript to completion. Patrick Riordan, Tim Reese, Debra Thrall, Akana Ma, Laura Santi, and Hannah Bonner all generously contributed their time and talents to the photography and illustrations. Thanks goes to Susan Cobb, Caroline Kutil, and David Lennon for their special efforts to bring the book to completion. My thanks also goes to Norman Bodek, President of Productivity, Inc. for his generous support.

In this book, if there is anything extraordinary, it is what I have received from my teacher. What is ordinary about it can be only my own addition.

I place this book at the feet of my great Acharya.

A.G. Mohan

YOGA FOR BODY, BREATH, AND MIND

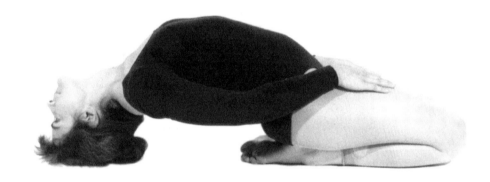

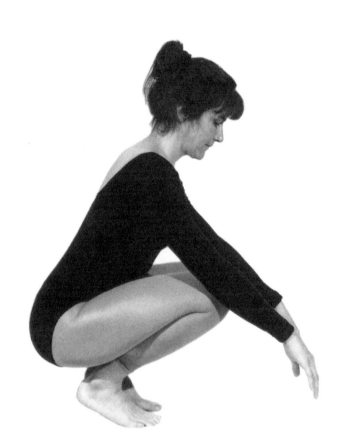

1

YOGA AND PERSONAL REINTEGRATION

Why Yoga for Personal Reintegration?

All of us have experienced times when it felt as though everything was coming apart, disintegrating around us into so many pieces, and we were without a way of holding them together. Yet often what is most fragmented and chaotic about the situation is not the events themselves, but the state of our own minds. On the other hand, we have also had occasions — albeit temporary — when we have experienced a state of integration. This is a state in which our minds perceive things clearly, when an underlying sense of order seems to prevail, and we feel full of a sense of love for everything around us. In short, we feel free.

We all wish to experience that state again. We even hope to find some way to actually *live* that way, instead of repeatedly falling into the clutches of our desire, anger, greed, frustration, sorrow, and despair. The fact that everyone around us would like the same thing is small consolation, and certainly no substitute for that deep sense of freedom.

Reintegration is the process of bringing us back to that state. It is the process of changing a wandering mind into a centered one, a wanting mind into a contented one, a self-indulging mind into a self-fulfilling one. It is a process called yoga.

There are various ways of describing what reintegration means, but they all stem from the same basis — that of a clear, unimpeded mind that sees clearly. As a result of seeing the people, things, and events in our lives as they truly are, we make decisions and take actions that lead in a positive direction.

We can also use the word *samadhi*, or "unity," to describe this state of integration. It is a state in which we are entirely absorbed or joined with the object of perception. No separation exists. In short, the state of integration is yoga.

This state of integration, or unity, is not something we create from scratch by diligent study or practice. At our center we are already integrated. We are all inherently capable of clear perception. The deepest state within us is always one of integration. Our minds are what mask that clarity, causing distortion and errors in action and judgment that lead to distress. An unintegrated mind leads to disease and bondage; the state of integration is one of radiant health and freedom. The reintegration of ourselves into that unified being which exists within us is unquestionably the highest of human goals.

All the means by which we see and experience the world are influenced by the contents of the mind. Because each of us is an individual, the means for reaching a clarity of vision will necessarily vary. Because we refine our perceptions by removing the obstacles that result from our personal character and experience, we must be clear about the specific nature of these impurities before we can decide upon the appropriate means for their removal. In order to be effective, any method of refinement must be shaped for the individual. That is, it must be personal.

In addition, only *you* can reintegrate yourself. Hence, the word "personal." Each of us might wish that we — or, better yet, somebody else — could simply remove the mind, wash it, and put it back so that suddenly we would have clear perception, but this is clearly not possible. Reintegration is a process of cleansing and removal that takes time, that must be personally relevant, and that can only be carried out by oneself.

The Yogic Approach to Personal Reintegration

True personal reintegration encompasses all elements in our lives. Accordingly, the yogic approach is an integrated one, in which all aspects of one's being will be touched. In fact, the very root meaning of the word yoga is "to integrate." These aspects include the body, breath, mind, food, the behavior of the senses, habits, society, and environment of the individual.

In order to reintegrate our minds we need to understand not only their relationship to these factors, but also the interconnection between them.

Integration is a matter of balance. Presently, many approaches exist for integration. Some consider the human system as a structure, while others consider it as a functional organism. These approaches use different methods for structural and functional integration. Some attempt psychological integration through mind work, while others use behavior modification

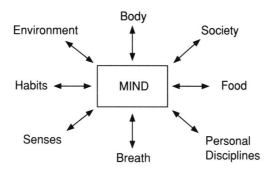

programs to bring about social integration. Used in isolation, these methods must ultimately be found lacking, simply because there is an interconnection between all the elements in the human system.

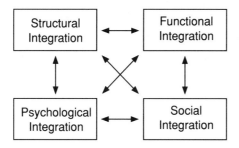

To work towards the state of integration, the path itself must be an integrated one. The practice of yoga is such an approach. It both uses and affects the structural, functional, psychological, and social aspects of the person. Yoga takes into account the present state of all areas of one's being and seeks to affect them all in whatever manner is most personally appropriate. Social integration comes about as a result of yoga practice and reintegration in other areas. When one's structural, functional, and psychological states are in order, social integration is assured.

The Problem: Mind — The Source of Misperception

The Bondage of the Mind

As human beings, we perceive the world through our minds. This would not present a problem if our minds actually perceived objects as they truly are. The mind, however, operates largely from a state of false understanding, often supplying us with inaccurate data. When we base our actions on this faulty information, we inadvertently create a great deal of suffering for ourselves and others. The crucial factor is the clarity of our perceptions. This is what determines whether we enter into a life of bondage or of freedom.

According to the philosophy of yoga, the mind normally moves in many directions. At the same time, we know that it is possible to direct all this movement, which suggests that some entity other than the mind is doing the directing. This entity we will call the Perceiver. The Perceiver itself is constant and unchanging. Just as the mind experiences the world through the senses, so the Perceiver "sees" through its own instrument of perception, the mind. It is what recognizes the movements and changes of the mind.

When the mind is not clouded over, or veiled, by the habits, tendencies, and associations it has accumulated over time, the Perceiver sees clearly. However, these other distorting factors are usually present, resulting in misperceptions, wrong actions, and painful consequences. The following illustration roughly captures this relationship:

When the mind is clear, we experience things as they truly are:

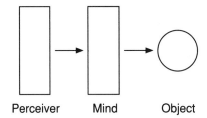

When the mind is not clear, our perceptions become distorted:

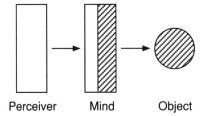

In the latter state, the mind is obscured by what the philosophy of yoga refers to as *kleshas*, or "impurities." It is as if the Perceiver must look through a dirty window. These impurities include the desire, hatred, fear, prejudices, reactions, and residues of our past experiences. They color and bias our perception of whatever we observe, so that when we look at a person, place, or thing through the windows of our minds, we see only the dirt. We don't see things as they really are, but as reflections of ourselves and our associations. The real problem arises when we identify with our minds and these distorted perceptions.

The Perceiver is inherently integrated. Its nature and its ability to see clearly do not change. It is in the mind that the lack of integration occurs, thereby affecting the perceptions of the Perceiver. When our perceptions are clouded, that lack of clear perception has the effect of disturbing our minds, body, and breathing. This sets up a kind of closed loop, in which lack of clear perception and disturbance to the system reinforce each other.

The foremost symptom of this situation is known as *dukha*, or "suffering." This is an uncomfortable feeling of restriction or oppression. The well-known stress syndrome of the modern world is one example of the result of this state, because most of us, when faced with the tension of unpleasant situations or environments, experience this sense of restriction or oppression. In short, we suffer. We may wish to get out of it, but insofar as it is a way in which we experience *ourselves*, where is there to go?

The Five States of Mind

As part of an effort to understand the mind and why it gets in the way of our freedom, it is useful to know that the mind can operate in a number of ways, and that there are five basic states of mind. The mind can change its focus — something like the way a person can switch the channels on a television set — or it can be directed to concentrate. In the first three of the five states, the mind is described as distracted; in the last two it is described as focused and voluntarily held on a chosen object.

1. The Agitated Mind

In the first state, the mind is agitated and out of control. The attention jumps from one thing to another in a hyperactive manner. It is almost as if the remote control button had gotten stuck, and the channels were continually changing on their own. When our minds are in this state, we are unintegrated.

2. The Dull Mind

In this second state, our minds are heavy and dull. We are in a state of mental inertia, such that movement and action are difficult. A person with a hangover, for example, is in this kind of state. In the mental television, the picture is hazy and unfocused.

3. The Distracted Mind

In the third state, the mind shifts its attention from one thing to another, but without the same kind of jumpiness as characterizes the first state. We alternate between being attentive and distracted, sometimes being attuned to one specific channel, and at other times flipping randomly between others. Due to this kind of fluctuation in our attention, the distracted mind still represents a state without integration.

4. The Focused State

In the fourth state, our minds are focused on a single object which can be either internal or external. The mental television now remains on one channel, and there is control over the focus.

5. The State of Absorption

This is the highest state, in which our minds are not merely focused on an object, but are so totally absorbed that it is like a pure, direct reception in which the television itself becomes unnecessary. The object is seen clearly, as it is, without any of our mental projections. No external force can disturb this focus, and in this state the mind is fully integrated. This is the state of yoga.

The Kleshas: Impurities of the Mind

We must also understand what the *Yoga Sutras* call the kleshas, or the impurities of the mind which we mentioned earlier, in order to reach the state of yoga or freedom. Although they may not be directly related to the object being perceived, they have a powerful effect on our perceptions and, therefore, on what we do. This makes them real. Indeed, according to yoga, anything that affects our actions is real and not an illusion. At the same time, even though it is real, it undergoes change. There are five kleshas:

1. False Understanding

When we see an object, we understand it as we perceive it, and not necessarily as it *is*. Unfortunately, we usually recognize our mistake only in retrospect. We start out believing that something is true, and through the outcome of our actions find that it is not — or vice versa. We can also start out believing something to be untrue, and come to realize that it was, in fact, true all along. Both represent a false understanding. The mind is therefore generally in a state that does not allow us to see or to accept reality as it is. This false understanding is the root klesha. The other four are all its by-products.

2. Mistaken Identity — The Ego

In this state, we identify ourselves with something that is not *us*. This identification can occur at various levels from things external to those internal to us.

3. Craving

We tend to recall the pleasant experiences in our lives, as well as the means by which they were created. If we continually want to repeat this same activity or obtain the agent that originally caused it, and if we mindlessly pursue these things, this is craving. When we feel such a need and are unable to fulfill it, we become disturbed. In the absence of the desired object, we are miserable. Thus, those people who have preconceived and mistaken notions of what constitutes comfort may spend their lives chasing the things they wrongly imagine will fulfill them. This, in turn, can only lead to dukha.

4. Hatred and Repulsion

This state is the opposite of craving. We remember negative experiences, and recall the agents and instruments that caused them. Consequently, we develop strong dislikes towards these things and try to avoid them. If we cannot do so, we suffer. In addition, when we hate a person or object, we may spend energy trying to affect them. This, again, is a form of misguided action, and one that is harmful not only to us, but to others.

5. Anxiety or Fear

Fear exists for all people. Indeed, it remains with us until our deaths, and expresses itself in various ways: We may be afraid to venture away from the security of where we now are; we may fear losing what we presently have; we may be afraid that something will happen to us in the future. The most basic fear, however, is the fear of death. Unlike craving or hatred, this state has no obvious cause. The symptoms consist of a state of anxiety, fear, or insecurity.

In the *Mahabharata*, an Indian epic, the question is asked, "What is the greatest wonder in the world?" The reply is, "Every day we see people entering the world of death, but the remainder still hope to live eternally. This is the greatest wonder on earth." The fear of death discriminates against no one; even the most learned people experience it.

Part of this fear appears to be related to our identification with our bodies, and our fear of parting with them. In other words, it emerges from our mistaken identity and our fear of losing what is actually not ours in the first place. It is only by knowing that one is the Self, and by remaining as the Self, that we go beyond this fear.

These five kleshas cloud our intelligence and knowledge, thus affecting how we act and, ultimately, the whole quality of our lives. However, the intensity of their effect varies. The kleshas can be subtle and hardly affect us at all, or they can be so intense as to blind us.

When they blind us, we are generally unable to find a lasting solution to whatever problem we face at the moment. Instead, our actions just become the pursuit of a way out. The escape routes we set up as a result then sever the connection between our minds and that to which we are relating. For example, when we feel that our egos have been injured, our minds may continue to rant and rave about the incident long after it has happened. We may resort to alcohol as a means of dissolving this connection.

Likewise, when we long for an object of pleasure that is not available to us, we may look for some substitute to gratify us. We may also use various drugs to sever our relationship with the unpleasant or painful experiences of the past. We may even go so far as to commit suicide to avoid intense fear or anxiety. (Suicide is often caused by a fear of life, rather than by the lack of a desire to live.) Ironically, another escape route may be meditation, when practiced without the proper guidance.

The kleshas work together to distract our perceptions and prevent us from seeing clearly. They cloud our vision, dirtying the window through which we gaze out upon the world. Therefore, to clean this window, we embark on the practice of yoga.

The Gunas: The Fundamental Characteristics of All Things

In addition to examining the different kleshas, the *Yoga Sutras* also explores the basic characteristics, or qualities, of the things that the mind observes and with which it interacts. All of life — including the mind itself — is composed of three such characteristics, called *gunas*. Therefore, understanding the gunas is important to understanding why the mind does not see things clearly. It is also important to understanding how the mind can be influenced to see clearly.

We said earlier that the Perceiver is constant and innately integrated. Yet everything we perceive in the world is constantly undergoing change. We could almost say that the single constant in our experiential life of the world is one of change, which comes about through the interaction of the gunas. Although the Perceiver is unchanging, and does not possess gunas, it must still perceive through the lens of the mind, which *does* have gunas and is extremely volatile.

Thus, we perceive according to which guna is most dominant in our minds. We infer that a particular guna is dominant in an event by looking at its effect on our perception. Therefore, understanding the gunas is important for understanding how the mind causes us dissatisfaction. The three gunas are:

1. *Satva*: This guna involves purity, lightness, clarity, stillness, tranquility, and pleasantness. It is represented by the color white.
2. *Rajas*: This guna produces excitement, passion, movement or agitation, and an intense drive to act. It is represented by the color red.
3. *Tamas*: The predominance of this guna makes one heavy, dull, and sleepy. Its lack of clarity leads to action without reflection. It is represented by the color black.

Although the gunas have fundamentally opposing qualities, they are all always present, working together in forming a person's nature, attitude, and potential. When one guna becomes more active, the others become less so. One replaces another. For example, when there is activity (rajas), there is no sleepiness (tamas).

One ancient illustration of this harmonious function between the three is the example of the oil lamp with a wick. The wick, made of cotton which is light and white, represents satva. The oil, which has the properties of movement and flow, represents rajas. The heavy basin containing the oil represents tamas. The three together produce the flame.

Thus, all three gunas are essential. In order for a person to function appropriately, however, the appropriate guna must predominate at the appropriate time. For example, we need tamas at night for sleep. When we must be active, we need rajas.

Disturbance, or dukha, is often caused when the gunas are not in accord with what we want or need to do. For example, we may feel sleepy in the morning, but need to be active, so we drink several cups of coffee. In the evening we need to feel sleepy, but may feel rajasic, and so resort to sleeping pills. In each case there is further disturbance both immediately and later, as a result of the attempted solutions.

That the gunas influence our minds and color our perceptions is made all the more complex by the fact that everything around us — including the five basic elements of Earth, Water, Fire, Air, and Space — all contains these three gunas. Therefore, our food and physical environment as well as our thoughts, breath, and intrinsic nature have an influence on our minds, depending on which guna is predominant in them.

Fortunately, this also means that these factors can be used to affect our minds in a positive way. Certain foods, breathing techniques, and so on, can be used to produce specific changes in the gunas. Appropriate action — that is, action which will lead us toward freedom — requires that we know how to use the gunas to our advantage.

The Solution: The Practice of Yoga

The word "yoga" has two roots. The first, *yuj*, means "to join." The unification of two things, whatever their nature, is called yoga. Some understand this to mean the joining of human and God, while others think of yoga as the hands joining the feet when one touches one's toes.

The second root related to the word "yoga" is samadhi. According to the *Yoga Sutras*, samadhi is the state of mind in which we voluntarily become so deeply joined with the object of our inquiry that the limits of our personal identity are temporarily set aside. When we are in such a state our perception is completely clear and we understand fully the thing to which we are relating (See Chapter 7, on Meditation).

The first root, yuj — "to join" — represents a process, or a means to an end; the second root, samadhi, represents a state of mind, which is an end in itself. Whether we want to touch our toes or reach God, there must be movement. This movement is yoga. If we reach the desired goal and stay there, that is also yoga. It may mean holding a posture or remaining in union with God. In either case, yoga is both the means and the end.

In Patanjali's *Yoga Sutras* (1:2), yoga is defined as the process of channelling the activities of the mind in the desired direction, and sustaining that focus without being distracted. As we said above, both the movement toward the goal, and the state of absorption itself, are yoga. Some have defined yoga in a negative sense as the restraining of the activities of the mind. However, the positive definition of yoga as "the directing of the mind's activities" presupposes that movement of the mind in one direction necessarily restrains it from going in other directions. For example, since you have chosen to read this book at this moment, you are not concentrating on something else.

As long as we identify with the mind and all that affects it, we are controlled by its inconsistent nature and its reactions to each new development within and around us. When reintegration happens, however, we cease to identify with the mind and remain as the Perceiver. Then the mind becomes the servant, rather than the master.

In this connection, yoga is often equated with one or another of the Hindu religious traditions, so it is important to clarify the difference between the two. While it is true that yoga emerged as a set of practices in an Indian religious context, it is not wedded to any particular religious tradition. Therefore, the practice of yoga is also used by various non-Hindu groups in India, as well as by some of the different sects of Buddhism throughout Asia.

Yoga talks about a process through which a person can attain freedom. At the same time, yoga is not about adopting any particular set of beliefs, but about coming to *know* through your own experience. It is not about becoming the blind follower of anything, but about assisting you on your own chosen path. There is nothing in yoga that competes with any religious orthodoxy or with any other system of belief. Rather, yoga is a vehicle for growth and development that anyone can adapt to one's own way of making life's journey. The emphasis in yoga is on doing and practicing, not on believing.

The broadest goal of your yoga practice is to reintegrate and clarify your vision. It is not concerned with the specific composition of that vision, but with learning to understand the nature of false perception and the ways to remove the obstacles. It is thus a process of elimination, not acquisition. In aiming to bring about personal reintegration, yoga is also about the pursuit of real freedom.

Obstacles on the Path Toward Reintegration

This journey toward reintegration is not without obstacles. Indeed, the *Yoga Sutras* (1:30) list nine major categories of things that can obstruct the sustained pursuit of reintegration: disease, heaviness, doubt, haste, exhaustion, temptation, illusion, stagnation, and regression.

Any of these experiences or attitudes, when acting upon the mind, can bring about the sense of restriction or repression we described earlier as dukha. We experience this as a feeling of disturbance in the body, breath, and mind. Nevertheless, on such occasions, it becomes all the more important to persist, as most of these obstacles are temporary.

In the face of such disturbances, it usually becomes difficult to discriminate clearly and to refrain from reacting to the people and events around us. This makes it hard to remain clear about our primary objective, our own reintegration. There are, however, several ways to calm down and return to a focused state — practical attitudes and actions that will support your efforts toward reintegration when the obstacles seem particularly overwhelming.

For example, when another person is successful, happy, and prosperous, the normal human tendency is to become jealous. This only leads to further distress, however, and prevents us from exploring the real challenges and possibilities in our own lives. It is better to be friendly and to share in the other's happiness. This creates a spirit of openness which allows us to bring out our own full potential.

When someone else is suffering unfortunate circumstances, it can be tempting to criticize. We rarely recognize the effect of doing so upon ourselves. It is better simply to be compassionate and show concern, resisting the inclination to find fault.

Likewise, when someone is performing a good action or seems motivated by a worthy cause, it is important to be supportive and helpful. On the other hand, if the other person is doing something which we feel is inappropriate, or which does not coincide with our own nature or values, we should step back and carefully observe before taking any action. If we ourselves are not in a state of clarity, our initial reaction may be wrongly motivated. When things get tense or heated up, we can also learn to use breathing techniques. Emphasizing the exhalation has a relaxing effect on the mind, and will help us to calm down.

In general, it is a good idea to reflect on the way your senses lead you to respond to events. Notice the control they exert on your reactions, thoughts, and perceptions. Often, without our being aware of it, they can be the cause of the problem.

It can help to reflect on the nature of life itself. Focusing on this kind of larger question and on the direction of our own personal lives can reorient us and thereby soothe our mental distraction. We can also get support from another source. Our difficulties often stem from various cravings in our minds (*raga*). We can reflect on someone who has confronted and overcome such desires and draw inspiration from their doing so, even asking ourselves, "How would this person I admire have solved this problem," or we may want to seek actual guidance from a teacher.

Sometimes it helps to investigate the nature of our sleep and dreams. Life, it is sometimes said, is but a dream. For example, when we examine the experience of deep sleep, we discover that it is a state without agitation. Exploring the nature of this experience may help us to attain a quiet state of mind during our waking hours. It is also possible to meditate or concentrate on an object of interest to you. You can choose anything that will engage your mind and reduce its disturbance.

Together, all of these techniques represent ways of detecting and responding to the obstacles to clear awareness. As you can see, they suggest that, far from being a set of abstract principles, yogic practice and training grow directly out of ordinary human experience. They recognize the kinds of experiences with which we all struggle, and attempt to provide ways with which to respond to them.

Action and Personal Reintegration

In addition to suggesting these specific ways of addressing and reducing the impact of the obstacles to reintegration, yoga also offers us a whole way of approaching our actions in the world. Action, after all, is a key element of life. There is no one who can escape acting. Our actions are significant, however, insofar as they either lead us into confusion and bondage, or into freedom. Some further our reintegration, while others do not. The difference rests in the state of mind with which we enter into the things we do.

In order for any of our actions to support our reintegration, including the practice of yoga, they must embody three qualities: refinement, reflection, and release. These three, together, are called *Kriya Yoga*.

Refinement

The Sanskrit word for refinement is *tapas*. *Tap* means "to burn or to cook." Like cooking, tapas is a process of refinement. The actions we undertake to refine ourselves — we could also say, to remove the kleshas, or impurities — are considered tapas. The yogic practices relating to physical disciplines and the training of the breath are two such methods. As we saw earlier in the discussion of the kleshas, the cleansing of these impurities from the mind is crucial to attaining the state of yoga.

Tapas is often translated as "penance, mortification, or fasting," for these practices can assist in the removal of the kleshas. These sorts of practices can generally be undertaken, provided they do not cause imbalance in the mind.

Reflection

If refinement is the burning that takes place, reflection is the fire that is used to cook or burn away our impurities. Reflection may involve the study of one's own religious or spiritual tradition; it may also include the study of such texts as the *Vedas*, the *Bible*, or the *Koran*. This kind of study helps in the process of self-understanding. For instance, we may read something in the Indian classic, the *Ramayana*, that elicits a response such as irritation, sympathy, or agreement. Such reactions arise from something within us, and can serve as an important starting point for self-investigation and reflection.

The practices of *asana* and *pranayama* — the training of our body and breath — can, as we shall see, also function as sources of reflection if they increase our knowledge of ourselves. This happens when we perform them correctly, that is, with attention and reflection. Indeed, it is important that we come to think of all our actions in this light, because any action done mechanically will become sterile and result in problems. Ideally, action and reflection should always accompany each other. This is why reflection is listed between refinement and release: Both require it in order to be effective.

Release

Sometimes, despite careful refinement and reflection in our actions, things simply don't turn out as we might have wished. To react to such results does nothing to further our reintegration. In fact, these situations call for just the opposite. Instead of reacting, we must learn to let go of our concern for the results of our actions. In other words, we learn to release our attachment to the outcome of each of our actions.

This doesn't mean that we don't establish and pursue goals. But sometimes our focus on our goals prevents us from simply attending to the quality of our action itself, regardless of the outcome. It is better to separate the goal — the outcome — from the action, and to function with detachment. This is especially important because it may actually turn out that we are pursuing an inappropriate goal. Reflection, along with a general attitude of release, will allow us to discover this more easily and to change direction. It is all too easy to spend a great deal of energy following irrelevant goals of little value. Moreover, if we attach too great a significance to a particular goal and are then unable to reach it, we may end up gravely disappointed and discouraged.

Surrender

Beyond release is surrender. If release is an attitude and an approach to individual actions, surrender is a total way of being. One of the ways that the *Yoga Sutras* talks about surrender is as surrender to God. It states that the seeker who develops a deep relationship of devotion and surrender with God will surely reach the state of yoga. The seeker must therefore accept God, trying to understand, praise, and seek God's help.

The *Yoga Sutras* speak of God as one who is beyond the false understanding and impurities that affect our own minds. He is the source of all knowledge, knowing everything to its full extent at all times. He is the first of all teachers and exists beyond time. God is the deepest essence of what we come to know through the practice of yoga. Surrender to God is therefore the process of opening ourselves deeply to knowing this reality, not holding ourselves back, or allowing ourselves to get caught up in all the things that distort our vision and misguide our actions.

The problem, when we do get caught up in these things, is that the fruits of our actions cause us to suffer. The residual effects of these experiences only cloud our perception further, so that we continue to repeat our actions mindlessly, never understanding their implications. This, of course, only leads to further suffering.

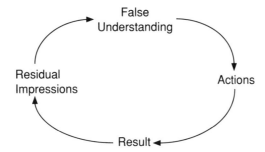

Surrender to God — the understanding and experience that there is something deeper at work in our lives — brings about a true understanding of ourselves. Although we might expect that prayers to God would help us to see God more clearly, Patanjali says that in doing this we will, instead, come to know ourselves better. For example, one practice that you can do is to sit down and repeat one hundred times the name of God that is most meaningful to you. Observe what happens to your mind in the process. You will probably notice that your mind travels to all kinds of places other than a focus on God. Indeed, you will be able to observe all your tendencies to distraction, as they come to the surface of your awareness. If you reflect upon these, you will come to understand more about yourself.

The path to clear perception takes time. We must know ourselves before we can know God. There are naturally problems and obstacles along the way — most of which exist within us — which hinder our progress in this endeavor. However, developing our understanding of surrender and our relationship with God will help us to refine our ability to reflect, and will eventually lead us into the clarity of vision which is the state of yoga.

The Eight Limbs of Yoga

We have seen that our experience of suffering happens as a result of our misperceptions and faulty understanding. We have also suggested that we find freedom when we are able to reduce these misunderstandings. The most basic tool for accomplishing this is discrimination, or the ability to distinguish between what will support our pursuit of freedom and what will not. The development of this awareness — which is also the key to our developing any clarity of vision — is, first of all, the recognition that we need to change. Secondly, it requires that we make the constant effort to cultivate such awareness.

The *Yoga Sutras* proposes a detailed method for developing discrimination and clarity (PYS II:29-55 and III:1-3). This method consists of eight parts, known as "the eight limbs of yoga." Together these eight limbs comprise a practical approach which addresses every aspect of one's being. They constitute an integrated process for removing the impurities that distort our vision, and give us tools with which to examine every facet of ourselves from all perspectives. Moreover, each of them is an arena in which we can also practice refinement, reflection, and release, all of which are directly related to the development of discrimination. These eight limbs are:

1. Yama

Yama concerns our behavior toward others and toward our environment. It includes deepening our understanding and practice of consideration, proper communication, non-covetousness, moderation, and the absence of greed.

2. Niyama

Where Yama involves our interactions with others, Niyama concerns our personal disciplines and our attitude toward ourselves. This includes personal cleanliness, contentment, the removal of impurities through discipline and proper habits, the continued learning about and acceptance of our limitations. Together, Yama and Niyama are concerned with our attitudes, which are extremely personal.

3. Asana

Asana concerns the use of the body, and is one of the primary subjects of this book. It will be discussed in detail in Chapters 2 and 3.

4. Pranayama

Pranayama is the practice of training our breath in ways that have an effect on our mind, our awareness, and our general state. It will be discussed in detail in Chapter 6. Both asana and pranayama are practical, and involve specific, teachable techniques. Pranayama is an aid to focusing the mind, while asana can also be a prerequisite to the practice of pranayama.

5. Pratyahara

Pratyahara addresses the influence of our senses on our minds when we wish to engage in specific actions. Ideally, the senses should faithfully follow the lead of the mind, instead of being drawn in many directions by the objects they are perceiving. Pratyahara is about withdrawing the mind from its servitude to the senses. This takes practice, as the responses of our senses can be difficult to recognize and understand.

6-8. Dharana, Dhyana, and Samadhi

These three concern training the activities of the mind. Dharana involves concentration, focusing the mind on a particular object. Dhyana stabilizes the mind in an uninterrupted state of concentration on the object. Samadhi, as we discussed earlier, is the pure awareness of the object — the mind free of its ordinary distractions and movements. This is the state of pure awareness and freedom. Together, these three limbs will be discussed in detail in Chapter 7.

The word *anga*, or "limb," is used to describe each of these areas of practice. Like the limbs of a tree, they develop simultaneously, rather than as sequential steps, even though in discussion they are arranged in an order that suggests movement from the gross to the subtle, or from external relationships to a refined state of introspection. In practice, however, the experience of each one informs the others at all times.

Often yoga is mistakenly identified either with postures or with sitting in meditation. A beginning student of the postures may feel that only these are necessary, while someone beginning to study meditation may feel that the postures are not useful. However, certain disciplines involving the body and breath are essential to support any meditation practice, while postures done without mental involvement and proper breathing will not lead a student into the full experience of personal integration. Moreover, as one's experience deepens, one comes to recognize the related importance of each of the other eight limbs as well.

As we will discuss in greater detail in the following chapters, one must learn to become flexible in both body and mind. This can be accomplished only by removing the obstacles at all levels of our being. Therefore, a properly integrated practice involves the unification of the body, the breath, and the mind, and must be done every day so that it becomes an integral part of one's life. Such a practice will then lead to the recognition and cultivation of all aspects of oneself.

A beginning student may start with any of the eight limbs. This is so, first of all, because we are all different, and different means are more or less appropriate starting points for each given individual. Secondly, however, if the right means are adopted, growth in one area will naturally lead to work in another, because all the areas are connected.

Suppose you are asked to look at yourself. Your understanding of this request can range from going to look at yourself in a mirror to sitting down and reflecting upon your own true nature. Yoga is the mirror that takes this variety of understandings into account through the eight limbs. It allows the student to begin at any level or in any area, depending on his or her present state of development. The first area one chooses is only the onset of the inquiry. Other directions will follow, even as the other areas develop, either at the same time or at some different point. Yoga aims at developing the total person in whatever manner is the most suitable.

The real issue, in order to begin and then to sustain our practice, is that we first recognize that our current understanding of how things are is false. We must accept that we need to take steps to change that understanding, and then have the real desire and willingness to do so. We must feel the strong need to travel toward the state of yoga, and then begin this practice, continuing on the journey without losing the spirit of the practice along the way.

The actual means we use are of secondary importance. They are provisional and may change. But our orientation and direction must be clear and consistent, for otherwise the actual mechanisms of our practice may become rote and meaningless. An authentic practice is to be done regularly, over a long period of time, and without interruption. We must undertake it with eager anticipation, optimism, and a positive orientation. Such a practice, whose longer range objective is kept clearly in mind, automatically enables us to practice detachment toward the events in our lives and prevents us from becoming disturbed by those forces which might otherwise distract us from our goals.

Practice and detachment are the means of travelling toward personal integration, or the state of yoga. Although some people may be born with this degree of clarity, the majority of us must engage in a sustained and sincere practice to reach this state and become established in it. According to the *Yoga Sutras*, faith in our goal gives us the energy to persist in the journey and to keep sight of that goal. It is the intensity of our yearning that brings about our full reintegration.

Aspects of Personal Reintegration

This book will explore in some detail three of the eight limbs of yoga: asana, pranayama, and meditation. These three are the practical limbs, and each of them is related to a particular aspect of personal reintegration. They are the starting point out of which the other limbs grow naturally.

Another way to look at it is that we are talking not about eight steps, to be followed in a linear order, but eight aspects of yoga. This is so, even though the arrangement of the eight limbs proceeds from the gross to the subtle aspects of our experience. There is, nevertheless, an internal unity among them; if the methodology adapted is as it should be, then all the aspects will naturally emerge in an organic unity, like the limbs of a tree. Moreover, together they will bring about the various aspects of personal reintegration.

The first of these, *structural integration*, is addressed by the practice of asana. Our bodies are structures that have been influenced since infancy by our birth, our movement patterns, our choice of work, the level of our activity, injuries, and so on. One's structure affects one's ability to function. A classic example of this is a backache. When you have a backache it becomes difficult to function well mechanically, so that even performing routine tasks such as sitting or lifting things becomes painful. Likewise, physiological functions such as normal digestion or breathing may be hindered. Moreover, the backache may leave you psychologically debilitated by depression, fatigue, and lethargy, all of which have social consequences as well.

Asana practice, the physical disciplines of yoga, reintegrate the body structurally. Using different movements and postures, the practice uses the physical body as the primary focus for integration. At the same time, out of respect for the connection between body, breath, and mind, asana practice incorporates proper breathing and mental concentration into these postures, in order to maintain a fully integrated approach.

According to yoga philosophy, structural integration truly occurs when the energy centers of the body, known as the *chakras*, are properly aligned. Since these energy centers are also connected to our emotional and psychological functions, integration of the one results in the integration of the others.

The second focus of this book involves *functional integration*. Yoga philosophy states that functional integration exists when the energy flow in one's system is in order. When our energy is focused we become centered and integrated. We can affect the state of this energy flow through what we eat, our personal disciplines and habits, the behavior of our senses, and particularly through our breath.

Pranayama, which deals with the breath, is one of the most important means of bringing about functional reintegration. In the process, it also leads to psychological integration. This practice removes impurities from the mind so that it is able to focus.

The connection between the mind and the body has been well established in Eastern thinking, and in some aspects of Western thought. The absence of *psychological integration* leads to structural and functional impairment, and vice versa. When the mind is disturbed, the body and breath become disturbed as well. Meditation techniques address this problem directly. In addition, various asanas and pranayama techniques assist in bringing about this kind of integration through the properly coordinated use of the body and breath.

Social integration is a natural result of these various practices and forms of integration. When our structural, functional, and psychological states are in order, we are able to engage in appropriate social interaction. It is something like the story of the army general and his nine-year-old son.

An army general once had a nine-year-old son who was quite bright and always asking questions. One evening, when the general was busy drawing up plans for war, the son came to him with more new questions. To occupy the child for a while, his father gave him a world map which had been torn into pieces, and asked him to set it right.

Expecting this to take the boy some considerable time, the father was astonished when his son returned in a matter of minutes, the map of the world restored. He asked his son how he had accomplished this so quickly, to which the boy replied, "It was very simple. I found that there was a picture of a person on the other side, and I put his pieces back together." With this, the father realized that when one sets the person right, the world will be all right. This is personal reintegration in its fullest sense.

2
ASANA — THE ROLE OF THE BODY IN PERSONAL REINTEGRATION

Asana is an obvious starting point for personal reintegration because it involves something concrete and tangible: the body. In almost any task, it is easiest to begin at the gross level and work toward the more subtle aspects. The same is true of reintegrating ourselves. For most people, the body is the primary object of which we are aware, so that most of us identify "Self" in some way with our physical being. We experience ourselves, our environment, and other people through our bodies. Consequently, the body is a natural place to begin the practice of yoga.

Appropriate asana practice — a practice incorporating body, breath, and mind — will strengthen, balance, and stabilize the body. As this happens our entire being will change in the same ways. Isolated development of one or two of the three areas cannot provide this. If we focus on the mind and breath only, for example, we will not be building a healthy body. An unhealthy body then becomes an obstacle to meditation or reflection. The integrated application of all three — body, breath, and mind — allows serious students to change, to outgrow limitations, and realize meaningful goals in their internal development and external lives.

The correct practice of asana will also help in balancing the structure and function of the chakras, the centers of energy in the body. As we change the position of the body in the various postures, we also move the position of the chakras. Each movement and configuration of the body, as well as of one's breath and emotional state, will have a different effect on these focal points of energy, thereby letting the body's energetic system balance itself. For the maintenance of good health, the correct alignment of the chakras and the ideal distance between them must be maintained. Proper asana practice with effective use of the breath will bring about this desired balance.

One important point of clarification before we proceed: Typically in the West, when people think of "yoga," they imagine these postures, or asanas. They assume that yoga is simply a discipline for maintaining a healthy body. This is, of course, a well-known result of asana practice. Properly planned and performed asana practice *will* enhance strength, flexibility, and endurance, and provide an unequaled sense of health and well-being. These goals, however, are by-products of the practice, not its ultimate or only aim. The physical orientation is simply one facet in the integrated approach toward one's total reintegration.

The Core Principles of Reintegration Asana

Nearly every school of asana has its own approach. Many schools emphasize mastery of final forms of the postures. The approach to asana we outline in this book is unique both in its emphasis and its simplicity. What is particularly powerful about Reintegration Asana is the underlying set of principles and the way these principles inform and direct the practice. This chapter will introduce you to some of these principles and elaborate on their practice.

1. Asana practice should be steady and comfortable, and make the body strong and flexible.
2. Asana practice should emphasize the spine.
3. Asana practice should be adapted to achieve your goal.
4. Asana practice should proceed in intelligent, orderly steps (*vinyasa krama*).
5. Asana practice should use the breath to integrate the body and mind.
6. Asana practice should use the breath to adapt postures.
7. Asana practice should use the breath for feedback.

Principle One: Asana practice should be steady and comfortable, and make the body strong and flexible.

In the *Yoga Sutras* (II:46) Patanjali defines asana as *sthirasukhamasanam*. *Sthira* means "firm, steady or alert," and is related to strength. *Sukha* means "pleasant" or "comfortable," and pertains to flexibility. Patanjali's definition is significant: Asana is not a specific posture, but rather a state. These qualities of steadiness and comfort apply not only to how our bodies should be, but to what our mental state should be as well. Asana is a state of attention without tension, that is accomplished by a movement or posture; it is an expression of the mind, body and breath working together in a balanced manner to achieve a balanced result.

The aim of a proper asana practice is the development of *both* strength and flexibility — a balance of sthira and sukha. Without both, you cannot move toward the larger goal of reintegration.

Principle Two: Asana practice should emphasize the spine.

Everything in the body is connected in some way to the spine. It is like the trunk of a tree: When it is strong and supple, the whole tree is healthy. When it is not, there is a greater risk of problems. So, improving the function of the spine develops a stable foundation for the entire body.

The soft tissue around the spine needs movement to keep the spine strong and flexible. The normal activities of modern life, however, don't involve much movement or, consequently, development of this area. Hence, back problems have become one of the biggest health problems in the modern Western world. The primary physical focus of an effective asana practice is therefore on the spine.

In Reintegration Asana, we emphasize the spine through three means:

1. selecting the right postures,
2. adapting the postures for maximum work in the spine,
3. and proper use of breath.

Principle Three: Asana practice should be adapted to achieve your goal.

Anyone practicing asana should begin with a goal or purpose. The goal may vary from day to day and from season to season. It may move from a specific goal, like the mastery of a particular posture, to a broad goal, like decreasing the stress in your daily life. In fact, each immediate goal in an asana practice is part of an ongoing movement toward the larger goal of total personal reintegration.

Having established both the immediate goal and the larger one, you will need to assess and adapt your practice continually to make sure it will accomplish these ends. The art of adaptation is how you accomplish this.

Principle Four: Asana practice should proceed in intelligent, orderly steps (vinyasa krama).

Vinyasa krama means intelligently placed, orderly steps. Once you have decided on your goal you need to determine how to get there safely and efficiently. To get anywhere, you must know the point from which you are beginning. Because each of us is different, the starting point of each person's practice will be different, even though our goals may be the same.

Herein lies the value of vinyasa krama in the path toward individual reintegration. This process takes into account each individual's starting point, specific characteristics, and limitations in mapping out the route to the goal. It bases that path on what is currently happening in your life, body, and environment, and thereby accurately determines the best means for you to reach your goal.

An attempt to reach a goal in one large step can often be disheartening and risky. If we break the goal into easy, manageable steps, we learn each of these steps thoroughly, and gain a sense of accomplishment at each step. This process also gives the student the chance to stop and evaluate at each step, make the necessary changes, and then proceed. This keeps both the path and the goal appropriately current with the constant changes within and around us. Moreover, we discover that the wisdom and practicality of this approach is useful in all areas of our lives. Change made in this fashion will be smoothly executed and suitable to each individual's personal characteristics, environment, and goals.

Principle Five: Asana practice should use the breath to integrate the body and mind.

Body, breath, and mind are intimately connected; a change in one is necessarily expressed in the others. When the mind is disturbed, the body and breath are affected as well. When the body is active, the mind and breath change their pace along with it. The power of this interaction is such that you can use all three to bring about the results you want. You can quiet your mind by quieting your breath; you can quiet your breathing by changing your activity. This is a key understanding in the practice of yoga, and will be discussed throughout this book.

Principle Six: Asana practice should use the breath to adapt postures.

You can adapt your postures to meet your needs simply through the use of the breath. The right time to inhale, the correct length of the exhale, and the appropriate use of suspension of the breath are all powerful tools that can make a practice beneficial or harmful. A posture done with a breath of four counts is different from the same posture done with a breath of eight counts. Holding the exhale while performing a movement can, under the right circumstances, strengthen the back. The retention of the inhale can *create* back problems when done incorrectly. Such is the power of breath to influence the outcome of one's practice.

Breath is a more subtle tool of adaptation, but it is also the most powerful. The breath acts as the greatest lever in the movement toward personal reintegration.

Principle Seven: Asana practice should use the breath for feedback.

The breath serves as a feedback mechanism for many aspects of practice. It is a particularly important indicator of sthira and sukha — of whether or not we are steady and comfortable. If our breath becomes short or labored, we are straining. This may indicate that a posture is too hard, that we are doing too many repetitions for our level of strength, or that we are straining inappropriately to overcome resistance.

Breath is also the main indicator of the focus of our attention. Since the regulation of breathing is critical to asana, when we find our minds wandering away from our breathing, we know that we are not concentrating, and no longer doing real yoga.

Ideally, the breath should be long, smooth, and under conscious control. Changes in the smoothness and length of breath indicate that our effort is no longer intelligent, and should therefore be modified. Essentially, such changes in breath signal the presence of resistance on the physical, mental, or emotional level.

Practice Guidelines

Know Your Purpose

As we discussed earlier, it is critical that you first determine your purpose in asana practice. This purpose may change from day to day, or it may stay the same until your needs change. Indeed, if you reflect vigilantly on your practice, its purpose *will* change as your life changes. For example, if your original practice was aimed at coping with a back problem you no longer have, you may find that you now want to build new strength and flexibility. Your routine will vary accordingly.

Before you begin, think about why you are taking up an asana practice. As you proceed, check with yourself again and again to see whether this original purpose remains your prime motivator. If it does not, evaluate *why* not, and reflect on what the new purpose of your practice might be.

Know Your Body

Since no two bodies are alike, no two bodies will look identical doing the same postures. Ideally, a teacher should adapt each posture and each asana routine to suit the needs of the student. In the ancient days, yoga teachers had one-to-one relationships with their students that entailed a sacred responsibility — to see to it that the student progressed without any long-term risk of physical or emotional damage. These teachers defined their role not only as one of teaching (*sikshana*), but also as one of protecting (*rakshana*) the student.

Basically, sikshana are the "do's," and rakshana the "don'ts," of asana practice. A good teacher should maintain the delicate balance between these two tasks of teaching and protection. A teacher too anxious about protecting may not allow a student to accomplish enough; on the other hand, a teacher too determined to reach a goal may bring harm. Thus, just as a balance between sthira and sukha is ideal, so is a balance between sikshana and rakshana.

One important point regarding the function of a teacher in this regard: It is the student's responsibility to have the right understanding when watching a teacher demonstrate a pose. When you first learn an asana, usually you will watch your teacher execute it, and then try it yourself.

There are advantages and disadvantages to this approach. Watching a posture will help you understand how to do it, but it can also fix an image in your mind of what the posture should look like. If you are not able to reproduce this picture with your own body, you may end up forcing the movement, getting frustrated and disappointed, and ultimately injuring yourself. At the very least, you may get a distaste for asana practice. Therefore, it is best to observe the teacher's work, keep a sense of detachment, and monitor your own experience of the pose. How it looks is of little consequence.

Even the most sophisticated teacher will not always have the right understanding of how much to work your body and how much to protect it. It will be up to you to determine the appropriate balance, and to change it when it becomes necessary. In the early stages of healing, for example, it is most important to err on the side of being too protective. At times, however, it is also important to overcome your resistance in order to make progress. At such times, working yourself is necessary. The best indicators of whether you are working too hard or not exerting yourself enough are the breath and your own heightened internal awareness, both of which we will cover in later sections.

Create the Right Setting

1. Generally it is best to practice indoors, so that the temperature is moderate and such elements as extreme wind or sun cannot disturb your practice. Pick a well-ventilated room with enough space for easy movement.
2. Use a carpet or padded surface for practice. It should protect your body from a hard floor, but be firm enough to provide support for balancing in standing postures. A surface with the qualities of sthira and sukha (firm and comfortable) will help you achieve these qualitites in yourself.
3. Clothing for asana should allow unrestricted movement and should keep you comfortably cool or warm, depending on the season and location.
4. If you play a sport or exercise before your asana practice, be sure to allow yourself some time for a rest before beginning your practice, so that your body, breath, and mind are fully available for use.
5. Eat lightly and allow at least one-and-a-half to two hours before your asana practice. If your stomach is empty, your diaphragm will move more freely, and your practice will be easier and more enjoyable.
6. Select the right length of time for your practice. This will depend largely on how much time you have available. You will also need to consider your preferences and stamina. The most important aspect is to sequence your practice correctly, so that you are adequately prepared, balanced, and rested. A regular fifteen-minute practice each day is far more beneficial than a two hour practice on weekends. It is better to do a short course thoroughly and with awareness, than to rush through a long complicated practice without the reintegration that makes it truly asana.
7. Select a time of day that works well for you. As in all aspects of practice, the time of practice must remain flexible, to serve your needs. Your work schedule, family responsibilities, access to suitable space, teacher availability, energy level, and how your body performs at certain times of day will all have some bearing on the optimal practice time.

   Morning is generally an ideal time for practice. To start your day with your body, breath, and mind integrated into an energized, relaxed and balanced state can have a positive effect.

However, a rigid adherence to this principle may have just the opposite effect. For example, a student who practiced in the early morning before work had an early plane to catch. It was cold when he got up at four in the morning to do his usual practice, which included inverted postures. By time he reached his destination later in the morning, he had acute back pain and a headache.

The body functions quite differently in the early morning when the joints have not been lubricated by use and the body is cold. If you practice that early, when it is still cold, you must modify your practice and devote more time to warming up. This is particularly true for those people with back problems.

If you have a hectic schedule, the only time you may be able to relax is before bed. This, then, would be the optimal time for you to practice. Your practice will need to be appropriate for sleep immediately afterward, of course.

The general guidelines are:

- Practice during a time when there is the least possible disturbance. You can then pay more attention to your experience and develop a sense of self-awareness that leads to reintegration.
- Relax during your practice. Make an effort to concentrate on your breath and movement, rather than the previous or subsequent activities of the day. This is difficult and demands constant awareness, but is well worth the effort.
- Be flexible in scheduling, but regular in doing your practice. Yoga is a process of continual change and growth. You will find that the assimilation of a practice into your daily life will yield extremely valuable results.

When to Interrupt or Discontinue Practice

Your constant observation and self-reflection will signal when a change is necessary. For example, when you practice certain postures every day to the exclusion of others, they may become addicting. It may be worthwhile to stop doing these particular postures, and to reflect, instead, on the factors that might be relevant in your attachment to them.

If you have physical symptoms such as those resulting from illness, rest may be more important than practice. In the case of injury, you may need to interrupt your practice to allow for healing. Often, in such instances, simple breathing exercises will accelerate your recovery.

Make Your Practice a Symphony

Asana practice should be a harmonious experience, never a struggle. The manner of breathing into a wind instrument — a flute, for instance — can create either a grating screech or a melodious song. The body, too, is an instrument. If used skillfully, as in the unison of movement and breath, the resulting posture is a useful and harmonious experience. When performed with the graceful orchestration of all its parts, asana can become a music of the body, breath, and mind. Such music moves everything it touches.

Putting the Principles Into Practice

Principle One: Steady and comfortable, strong and flexible.

Steadiness and comfort (or sthira and sukha) are functionally related. If a person is stiff when sitting on the floor, he or she won't be able to focus attention on, say, a breathing exercise. He or she will not have sukha, flexibility, and therefore will not be able to function with the steadiness of sthira.

Conversely, a very flexible student may become so comfortable in a particular posture that his or her attention will wander while performing it. Neither of these cases is truly asana, as each lacks the characteristics by which it is defined: sthira and sukha.

The key to effective asana practice is a balance between building strength and developing flexibility. An imbalance between strength (sthira) and flexibility (sukha) may create problems. Quite often asana is mistakenly seen simply as a method for increasing flexibility and relaxation; the aspect of strength is entirely overlooked.

If you become flexible without becoming strong, many postures involving the back become ineffective. Indeed, you can accomplish the final form of the posture without using the back at all. You may even do the final pose in a way that may harm you. Although the posture may *look* good, it may also be straining the body in a dysfunctional way.

Any structure will give way at the point of least resistance — too much flexibility leads to too little resistance in some areas. You may achieve a posture not out of a balance between strength and flexibility, but because your body is giving way at a weakened or overly flexible point. Eventually that area may become overused and injured.

A person with great strength and limited flexibility is in equal jeopardy. For those with limited range of motion, even a simple movement may cause pain or even injury. Just bending over may become a problem, and any spontaneous unusual motion can notably increase the risk of injury. In addition, chronically tightened abdominal muscles can inhibit circulation and visceral movement, thereby inhibiting digestion and the vitality of the organs in the lower torso.

On the other hand, in the overly flexible student, it is as if the upper and lower parts of the body become functionally disconnected. One part can work without relation to the other simply because of this kind of flexibility. Eventually, this imbalance may result in back problems. The back problems, in turn, will affect the "front" or lower abdominal area, causing problems with digestion, the menstrual cycle, and so on. A weakened muscular system is often a major factor in problems such as a hernia or a prolapsed uterus.

The importance of balance holds true for the amount of exertion in an asana practice as well. Without adequate movement the body becomes stiff, perhaps even painful. But too much exertion may also cause pain or injury. An appropriate asana practice includes the right amount of work at an intensity that challenges, but does not injure or fatigue, the student — again, the balance of steadiness and comfort.

The *Yoga Sutras* (II:50) describe the means for achieving sthira and sukha as fourfold:

- Intelligent or proper effort (*prayatna*).
- Recognition and reduction of resistance (*shaitilya*).
- The proper use of breath (*ananta*).
- Identification of one's aim, purpose, or goal (*samapatti*).

Overcoming Resistance through Intelligent Effort

All movement, whether it be physical, mental, or emotional, involves effort and encounters resistance of one sort or another. In asana it is vital that you recognize the resistances that may prevent you from practicing correctly. All movement involves friction; therefore, it is important to determine precisely what and where that friction is. Resistance can be physical, mental, or emotional, and can involve the body, breath, and mind.

For example, let's say you want to do a strong seated forward bend, such as *paschimatanasana*. Your resistance to it might originate in physical limitations — stiff back or legs, emotional resistance, the fear of bending forward, or some combination of the three. A good teacher will watch how your body works in the preparatory postures and in the final posture itself, and will adjust your program to ensure that your effort is intelligent and proper, rather than forced.

One common danger of a yoga practice occurs when students ignore their limitations and force themselves into a pose. This is not to say that a student absolutely *cannot* do a posture he or she wishes to do — it is only to say that such postures should not be forced initially. Once you recognize your limitations, you can adapt the posture in a variety of ways: You can vary the intensity, change the breathing, repeat the posture, or limit the duration of time that you stay in the pose. The thing to remember is that force will only provoke resistance. A practice should be like filing rather than chiseling.

Overcoming Resistance through the Proper Use of Breath

The importance of breath in any context cannot be overemphasized. Breath is life, and asana without proper breathing is not useful either in terms of personal reintegration, or of true yoga. The Sanskrit word ananta has various meanings, including "that which is endless." In the context of asana it means "breath," because breath is endless, coming into the body when we are born and leaving it only when we die. What gives a body life is the breath.

Breath functions in a multitude of ways. The state of your breathing will instantly reflect resistance and is therefore an effective means of discovering and monitoring it. The breath also indicates how hard you are working, demonstrating whether or not you are pushing beyond your limits. It is also a means of focusing the mind, which is a prerequisite state for effective asana practice.

In addition, breath can be a means of reducing resistance. For example, when you practice *paschimatanasana* (seated forward bend), you can circumvent the resistance created by a stiff back or hamstrings by exhaling smoothly as you release your torso forward over your legs. This is also a safety device — it is not possible to force your body beyond its limits if you focus on the quality of your breath throughout your practice.

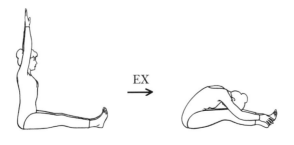

EX
→

To summarize, for an effective asana practice that results in steadiness and comfort, and strength and flexibility, consider the following factors:

- Understand and appreciate the connection between your body, breath, and mind.
- Evaluate your resistance to the proposed practice in terms of your body, breath, and mind.
- Use your breath to recognize and reduce resistance, to evaluate the intelligence of your effort, and to determine whether you are accomplishing your aim.

Principle Two: Emphasizing the spine.

We emphasize the spine through selecting postures that work the spine, and through adapting those postures to maximize our effort in that part of the body. To accomplish the former, we recommend working with the twenty asanas explained in this book. To accomplish the latter, you must become practiced in the use of awareness, breath, and movement for adaptation.

Awareness and Adaptation to Emphasize the Spine

In each posture, movement, and breath, be aware of the role of the spine, and notice the amount of movement or effort needed in the back. You can maximize the movement in the spine by positioning the rest of the body in a way that allows the spine to move easily. Generally, this involves a softening of the arms, neck, and legs that will release tension in these areas, and allow the work or focus to be transferred to the spine.

Let us look at this concept more closely. There is a significant, qualitative difference between raising your arms in a relaxed way, and raising them when they are stiff and straight. Lifting an already straightened and stiff arm allows for little movement in the spine, and tightens the neck and shoulders. On the other hand, movement that begins at the center of the body (in the torso) and progresses to the extremities actively involves the spine and avoids any tension in the neck and shoulders.

As an example, try this arm movement on your own, paying attention to your torso: While your arms are at your sides, first straighten them; then, keeping them stiff throughout the movement, bring them overhead, either by raising them to the sides or in front of you. Repeat this a few times.

Next, keeping your elbows, wrists, and hands relaxed, begin the arm motion again. This time, when raising your arms, begin with the elbows slightly bent, then gradually straighten them during the movement, finally extending them as the movement ends. Allow your torso to move as well.

Repeat this a few times, noticing the different quality in the areas of muscular involvement.

Using the Breath to Emphasize the Spine

Intelligent use of the breath also works the spine. The practice of inhaling and exhaling with the appropriate movements will heighten your awareness of the spine and bring more emphasis to it in the practice of each asana.

Principle Three: Adapting your practice to achieve your goal.

Establish the Purpose of Your Practice

Know the purpose of your practice before you begin each session. Examine how this purpose fits in with your larger goal of reintegration, and make the changes that will keep this immediate goal consonant with the practice. For example, if you have had a stressful day, your goal for an evening asana practice may be to calm down. On the other hand, you may wish to design your practice to wake up your body and mind in preparation for evening activities. To know your purpose, you need to reflect on how you feel in the moment and how you would like to feel at the end of your session.

You must continually redefine your practice on an ongoing basis, to insure that your goal is realistic and the course for achieving it appropriate. It is easy to fall into habits, especially with regular or daily activities such as asana practice. When this happens the practice may become sterile, and the sense of vitality and progress may disappear. The mind wanders, focus on the body and breath is lost, and what was originally asana practice becomes simply a set of mindless exercises.

Adapt Your Practice to Meet Your Goal

Any practice aimed at improving yourself must reflect the constant flux of daily life. Each day, your body, mood, schedule, environment, and so on, will differ. In light of this, on certain days a longstanding goal or practice may require some reflection or change. You accomplish this change through adaptation of both your practice as a whole (the specific poses you put together), and the poses themselves. This is the art of adaptation — a subtle and complex art best learned with a qualified teacher.

Let us take the example we talked about above. On the evening of a stressful day, the routine you design to calm you down may be quite different from the routine you design to wake you up early in the morning. Postures that center the body would be used in the evening, while postures that energize would be used in the morning. However, this is not the whole story.

It is possible that you might use the identical set of postures in the evening as in the morning, but with a different emphasis of breath and movement. You could accomplish entirely different ends by adapting the same postures. This is because no specific asana has a precise, intrinsic purpose. Rather, its form should be adaptable enough to serve an individual's specific needs.

Important adaptation principles include the following:

Adapt the postures so that you emphasize function rather than final form. Despite people's tendency to assign a general purpose to particular asanas, there is no standard intrinsic purpose for any asana. People hope that one posture will be the cure for a sore lower back; another, the remedy for constipation. In fact, while a posture may have a certain *function*, such as to stretch the back, the posture's *effect* will vary according to the body, the movements, the age, psychological state, and lifestyle of the student. The effect will also vary according to how the student performs the posture.

All asanas have a name, form, and characteristics. For example, paschimatanasana (seated forward bend) is the name of a posture, which has a particular form, and whose function is to stretch the back. The characteristics describe this function, and are therefore its most important aspect. So, you adapt the form for the individual, in order to preserve this intended function at a given point in his or her practice.

Unfortunately, quite often a student's only goal in asana is to achieve the final form of a posture. In trying to copy an ideal form, he or she frequently distorts or loses its real function. This forcible distortion is counterproductive to one's progress and, in fact, should not occur in any aspect of yoga. Asana should not simply be an external form into which you fit your body, but should arise from within you. What you see in the mirror is the form. What you *feel* is the function of the posture. Unity, not uniformity is the goal of yoga.

This is only natural since uniformity is not what we observe in people. People differ on many levels, so their needs and priorities will necessarily be different. The vast spectrum of body types and conditions assures that any particular posture or movement not only will, but should, look different in every student. Therefore, imitation of another person's position in an asana is not relevant to one's own purpose and may, in fact, be counterproductive or harmful. The adaptability of postures makes asana different, but useful, for all people.

Recognize resistance and use adaptation to reduce it. Adaptation is based largely on the recognition and reduction of resistance. A student or teacher must determine the areas of resistance, and then adapt the movements and positions so their function is no longer hindered or changed by the resistance.

For example, two students — one with flexible hamstrings, hips and back, and another with stiffness in those same areas — require very different versions of paschimatanasana (seated forward bend) if that posture is to produce its desired effect. If the two were to attempt the identical posture strictly according to a pictured ideal, the flexible student might derive no benefit from it and the stiff student might hurt him- or herself, or, at the very least, find the experience uncomfortable and frustrating.

In other words, you must redesign the posture both to achieve comfort and stability, and to fulfill its intended function. Rigid adherence to the ideal form is simply habit or conditioning, whereas adaptation to insure function is an act of creativity.

In addition to physical resistance, other types of resistance can affect your practice and must be considered in planning a course. Your mental and emotional state in general, and with regard to asana itself, are major components in a well-conceived asana practice. Physical activity without careful consideration of these factors yields only limited results in terms of the larger context of yoga. All facets of your being must be included in any movement toward wholeness.

Find the guidance of a qualified teacher. Careful adaptation of postures to suit the individual is imperative. The guidance of a qualified teacher is essential for this. A good teacher will help you to understand your purpose and to adapt routines so that the functions of the asanas, and not the final external forms, remain the first priority. Only in this way is a student truly doing yoga.

Principle Four: Vinyasa Krama — orderly steps toward a goal.

Any student appropriately using the adaptation process described above is practicing vinyasa krama. For example, if your goal is to master a difficult backbend, and you choose to accomplish it by working first on gentler backbends, you are taking the step-by-step path that is vinyasa krama.

There are, of course, many ways of accomplishing most goals. In asana, too, there are many different vinyasa kramas for each posture. The differences may center around the physical characteristics of the students, the limitations or resistances involved, or the intention of the postures. A single posture can have entirely different effects, depending on the sequence leading up to it. The effects of adhomukha shvanasana (downward dog) and paschimatanasana (seated forward bend) for example, will vary with each different vinyasa krama leading up to each posture.

Three Sequences for Seated Foward Bend (Paschimatanasana)

1.

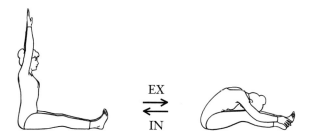

2.

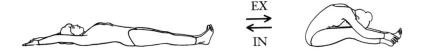

3.

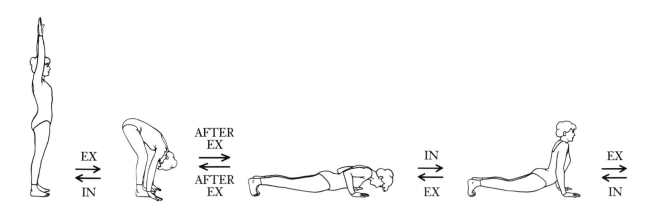

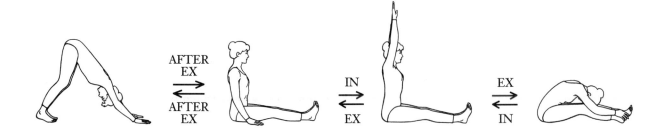

Three Sequences for Downward Dog Pose
(Adhomukha Shvanasana)

1.

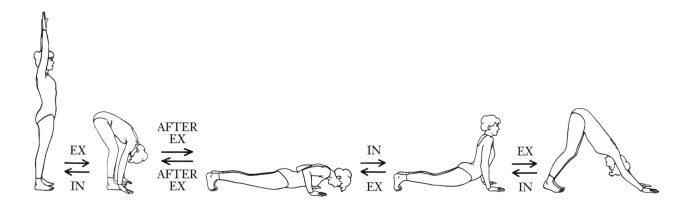

2.

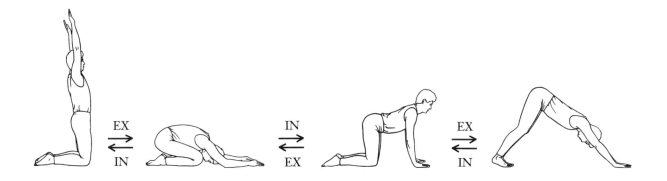

3.

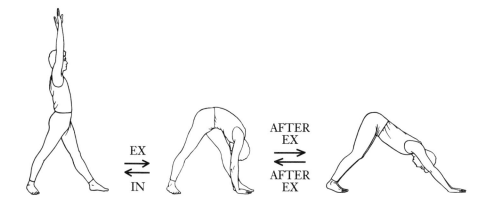

You can see from the above examples that vinyasa krama is an art. Simply doing easier versions of a posture to prepare for the final posture is a good place to start, but may not suffice to bring about the intended effect, and may not address the needs of the individual. Designing vinyasa krama is best done with the guidance of a capable teacher.

The Role of Static Postures in Vinyasa Krama

Since the word asana also means "to stay," some schools of yoga propose that all postures must be executed by staying in them for long periods of time. Also, most asana books describe only the final posture, without pictures or descriptions of its preparatory stages. As a result, students often attempt only these final postures, and work to stay in them for extended periods.

Strictly speaking, there can be no true "staying" or stillness in a posture because all of asana is controlled by the breath, and correct breathing involves movement of the body. Even postures held for some specified time involve the motion initiated by the breath. This state is a dynamic stillness rather than an absence of movement. Thus, the staying should be the result of movement, and in it the desire to move should disappear.

The prerequisite for getting to any final posture or destination is the movement that was necessary to get there in the first place. Staying can't exist without some prior movement. You must know how to move in order to know how to stay; you must know how to use movement and breath together correctly in order to hold a position in which both are comfortable. Only then will you attain the benefits of staying. Otherwise, staying can be a forced contortion of the body, and will have none of the beneficial aspects of asana. You will sometimes be able to recognize when you are forcing a pose as opposed to practicing asana correctly by paying attention to your breath — a topic to be covered under the following three principles.

If you approach the concept of staying in postures in this manner, your experience at the final stage will be a pleasant and useful one. Many students who assume that postures must always be held, and therefore begin learning them in this way, become frustrated and discouraged. They most certainly have to work too hard and, sadly, may never feel the positive effects of a stationary but comfortable asana.

Principle Five: Integrating the body and mind through the breath.

Breath is the bridge between the body and the mind. It is to the body what thought is to the mind. Thought moves in the mind as breath moves in the body. We need only observe the holding of the breath that accompanies fear, the quickening and shortening of it in anger, or the smoothing of it in relaxation, to realize the mind's immediate and powerful effect on our respiration. Equally clear is its effect on the body when, for example, an upsetting phone call at dinner instantaneously reduces a ravenous appetite to the inability to eat anything at all. Obviously, a change in one area produces some change in another. This relationship is constant and immutable.

The primary focus of your asana practice must be on the unity of the body, breath, and mind. Direct your attention to the connection of the body and breath, so that as your body moves into a position, your mind focuses on the correct breathing for that particular movement. To do so, your mind must observe the speed and direction of the movement, recall the appropriate breathing pattern, and adjust the breath accordingly. In this way, your body, breath, and mind come together in accomplishing a single activity. This integration of purpose is yoga.

Become Aware of Your Breath

Although our breathing goes on continually, most of the time we are not conscious of it. By becoming conscious of the components of the breath — noticing when we inhale, exhale, and hold or suspend our breath — we link our minds with our breathing.

Take a few conscious deep breaths now. Simply notice where you breathe more fully: in the chest or in the diaphragm. Notice whether the inhalation or exhalation is longer. See if you can smooth out your breath.

It is imperative that this same awareness of the breath, this linking of the mind and breath, be present throughout your entire practice of asana. Your breathing should be a conscious, slow, and comfortable process using the chest and diaphragm fully.

There are many patterns of both conscious and unconscious breathing. We breathe quite differently when we sleep, run, think, or lift a heavy weight. There are also many ways to breathe in asana, each appropriate depending on the student, situation, and purpose of the practice. Any breathing pattern, however, automatically involves movement of the body, primarily the spine and torso.

Movement and breath have a cause-and-effect relationship. Movement causes breath, and breath causes movement. When we move the body, as in walking, dancing, or any other physical activity, our breathing pattern automatically changes. The rate, depth, and evenness of inhalation and expiration will adjust to reflect the intensity and familiarity of the movement. Likewise, the act of breathing itself causes motion. Notice, for example, the movement of your diaphragm, ribs, spine, and shoulder girdle as they expand and contract the torso to accommodate the changing volume of air in your lungs. The two are inextricably linked.

Take a deep breath and notice the movement in your spine. To some degree all breathing includes this movement, but most asanas involve using the spine to an even greater extent. When used correctly the breath can easily and naturally facilitate that movement.

Ideal Methodology of Breathing

In asana, ideal breathing involves both the chest and abdomen, and is deliberately used to move the spine in ways that enhance each posture. As the inhale begins in the upper chest, the spine naturally straightens or arches slightly. An easy, controlled inhale should begin in the chest, lengthening the spine just to the point where the diaphragm barely begins to suck inward, but not so far that the abdomen is drawn inward. This portion of the breath keeps the spine erect, supporting the body for effective alignment in postures. Exhalation during asana should be initiated by gently contracting the lower abdomen and diaphragm. It is a healthy use of the lower abdominal muscles.

The process of inhaling first into the upper chest, then into the lower chest, extends the upper spine. Beginning each exhale with the lower abdomen lengthens the lower spine. In this way the entire spine is moved by the breath. Combining the appropriate part of the breath with particular movements naturally facilitates these movements. For example, inhaling into *shalabhasana* (locust) naturally arches the upper torso into the position. Exhaling on forward bends automatically helps fold the body.

During asana it is important that the breath remain relaxed, holding no tension. (Note that a common sign of tension — occurring spontaneously in fright or when one is exerting great effort, for example — is holding the breath.) Ideally, therefore, one's breathing during asana should be smooth, slow, and steady. Speed can be misleading because, despite being outwardly impressive, it may be less demanding than slow motion.

In general, quick activity allows the mind to wander; an event is over before the mind can do anything about it. An action done with awareness and control, on the other hand, requires sustained attention throughout its entire duration. This focus, the linking of the body, breath, and mind during a series of movements or postures, is the main priority in asana. The interaction of your body and breath sets in motion the process necessary for transformation. If your entire being is involved, the movement or posture will have a much greater impact.

One method for linking the body and mind through movement and breath is to make your breath encompass your movement. Begin the breath an instant before you actually initiate the movement, and extend it just slightly beyond the actual completion of the movement. For example:

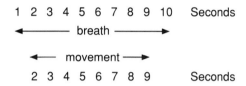

In this way your breath and movement are ideally coordinated. In the process, you engage your mind and breath with the movement. Your concentration assures that your mind is dynamically involved in the present, so that your goal of integrated activity can be accomplished.

Ujjayi or Throat Breathing

The breathing you should use in asana is called ujjayi breathing. This is a method of controlling the flow of air in order to regulate the length of the breath. It is done by slightly closing your throat so that the breath makes a sound just loud enough to hear. You will also feel it in the back of your throat. Consequently, this type of breathing is called "throat breathing." Try this breathing first on the exhale as it is easier than with the inhale, which tends to be a little rough or jerky when first attempted.

An important benefit of this type of ujjayi breathing, in addition to the control it provides, is that its sound can be used as both a feedback mechanism and an object of concentration. The nature of the sound and the changes in it immediately indicate to the student the presence or absence of sthira and sukha. More importantly, keeping one's awareness on the breath automatically links the mind and breath.

Principle Six: Using breath to adapt postures.

As we have said, any movement of the body provokes breath, and breath necessarily provokes movement. It is important to recognize that each type of movement has a specific breathing pattern that most easily and naturally accompanies it. For example, it is easiest to lift the arms above the head on the inhale, because this movement automatically expands the upper chest. Likewise, it is easiest to bend forward at the waist on the exhale, as the movement compresses the lungs, forcing the air outward. Although some exceptions occur, inhaling facilitates most opening or lengthening movements, while folding or bending movements are best done on the exhale.

Generally, the body-breath linkage follows these principles:

1. Raising the arms involves inhalation. Lowering the arms involves exhalation.

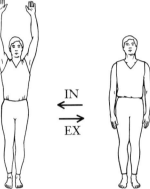

2. Bending forward involves exhalation. Returning to standing involves inhalation.

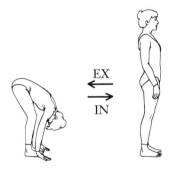

3. Twisting involves exhalation. Returning to a forward position involves inhalation.

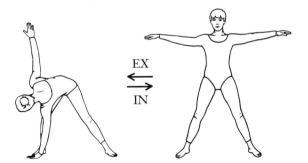

Another important aspect of breathing you can add to asana after you understand (and practice) the above concepts is the holding of the breath after you inhale and exhale. Try holding after the exhale first, as this is the easier and safer of the two. The power and myriad subtleties of the breath that are revealed by this type of variation can add a new dimension to any posture or practice as a whole.

In asana, use ujjayi breath on both inhale and exhale, doing chest to belly breathing. Your breath should remain consistently smooth, slow, and relaxed. In this way, it can function as a feedback system and a method for focusing the mind. This level of synchronized movement and breathing will greatly intensify and enrich the experience of asana practice, and is definitely a goal worthy of diligent pursuit for experienced, healthy students.

Outlined below are several additional ways to use the breath in adaptations of asana:

1. Alter the length of the inhale, the exhale, or both.
    *   If you are very strong, increasing the inhalation will have a strengthening effect.
    *   Increasing the exhale in forward bends may have a releasing effect that enhances stretching.
2. As discussed above, retain the breath after the inhale, suspend it after the exhale, or both. This will intensify the effort necessary in most cases.
3. Use the breathing opposite to what is customary (e.g., arching on the exhale).
4. Use the breath continually as an observation tool indicating effort and resistance.
    *   A shortening of breath is a signal to change the intensity or modify the posture so that body, breath, and mind remain balanced and work together at the optimum level. (For examples, refer to the discussion of *uttanasana* in Chapter 3.)

Abilities related to inhalation and exhalation vary widely among individuals. Some people are able to easily extend inhale, but not the exhale, or vice versa. Ideally, the inhale should equal the exhale, so that often a goal will be to focus on cultivating the capacity for one of the two breathing components.

You can concentrate on lengthening either of these components by allowing the easier one to be free, gradually extending the other over a number of breaths. Or you can fix a minimum duration for the more difficult component — say, six seconds, for example — keeping that part of the breath consistent and allowing the other to be unmeasured.

As we discussed above, the spine also has a considerable influence on the breath. Restrictions in the spine can cause restrictions in your breathing. Of course, the reverse is also true — you can develop your breathing capacity by using postures that facilitate the specific part of the breathing pattern that needs more work. Using postures that arch the upper spine will open your chest and facilitate inhaling. Postures that emphasize use of the diaphragm will be helpful for students who have trouble exhaling.

Principle Seven: Use the breath as a feedback device.

The sound and feel of your breath can furnish a lot of information about what you are doing. In asana it can provide feedback about the amount of effort you are using, whether the speed and range of motion are appropriate, and whether or not you are operating within your own comfortable limits. It is important to let the breath be an indicator of when to stop and start, how much is too much, and so on.

This is done by remaining aware of your breath and keeping it smooth, long, unforced, and comfortable. A change in any of these qualities is an indicator that you should work less intensely, lessen the speed or range of movement, rest until your breath returns to normal, or perhaps end the practice. In other words, use your mind and breath as a feedback for fine-tuning your practice to your own body and its needs. Based on this system, the adaptations you make will keep your practice a meaningful one.

Your first priority is your ability to take complete breaths. When the breathing cycle (a full inhale and exhale) is not completed, you will feel resistance and inhibition in your movement. Most important is that you be able to exhale smoothly and completely for a comfortable length of time. Holding the exhale too long increases pressure in the stomach or other areas; holding your breath after you inhale will create internal tension, increasing pressure in the neck and head that will cause discomfort and other difficulties. Therefore, the length of each breath should remain comfortable throughout each full cycle.

The length of breath and movement should also be comfortably matched. For beginners, if the breath becomes short, uneven, or panicky the movement should either be shortened to accommodate the breath, or accomplished in two separate movements, each with its own full and comfortable breath.

3
THE ASANAS

Hundreds of different postures (asanas) are practiced by yoga students and teachers, and hundreds of descriptions can be found in the literature of yoga. This tremendous variety, together with the many options they provide, make asana a truly accessible, enjoyable, and useful form of yoga. It is practiced throughout the world by people of various backgrounds, ages, physical conditions, and levels of expertise, and has been highly esteemed for thousands of years.

Due to the great adaptability of asanas, you can use a single posture to fulfill various functions just by modifying it. By adapting the following twenty postures you can achieve almost any purpose relating to the body. You will need to use the breath correctly, recognize and reduce resistances, and adapt the aim of your practice as it evolves. With this approach, twenty postures will suffice to provide everything necessary for the structural development that ultimately leads to a state of balance and clarity.

Each of the twenty postures has many functions, variations, and possibilities for adaptations. We will give some of these for many of the postures, but will only go into detail on the standing forward bend (uttanasana). It is not within the scope of this book to adequately cover the infinite possibilities of all the postures. To be truly accurate, each asana must be individually altered for each student, at each practice.

The classical form of each asana has been described for your information. The vinyasa krama to reach the classical form has to be learned from a teacher over a period of time. Each asana includes a choice of balancing postures to be done after completing the pose.

We have presented the following categories of information:

1. The Classical Posture: The ancient texts on yoga describe only the final or classical form of the postures. The relevant preparatory poses and orderly steps (vinyasa krama) required to reach the final form have to be learned from the teacher. The classical form of each asana has been described for your information.
2. The Modified Version: A modified version of the classical posture for the "average healthy individual" is included.
3. Vinyasa Krama: A vinyasa krama for the modified version of each posture has been included.
4. Other modifications are given where relevant.
5. Special notes, if any, are included whenever appropriate.
6. Balancing Postures: A choice of balancing postures for each posture is given.

Please note that the categories of information for each pose may vary and are not exhaustive.

Complete List of Asanas

1. *Samasthiti* (Standing Pose)

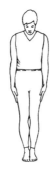

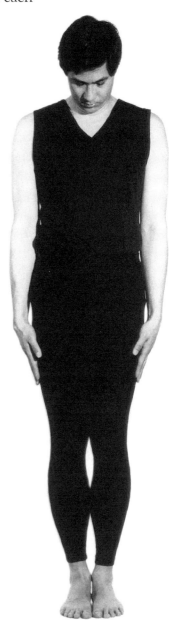

2. *Parshva Uttanasana* (Asymmetrical Forward Bend)

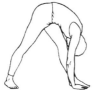

3. *Uttanasana* (Standing Forward Bend)

4. *Ardha Uttanasana* (Half Forward Bend)

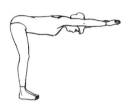

5. *Ardha Utkatasana* (Chair)

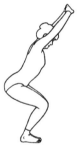

6. *Utthita Trikonasana*
   (Standing Twist and Lateral Bend)

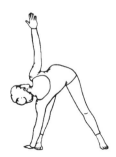

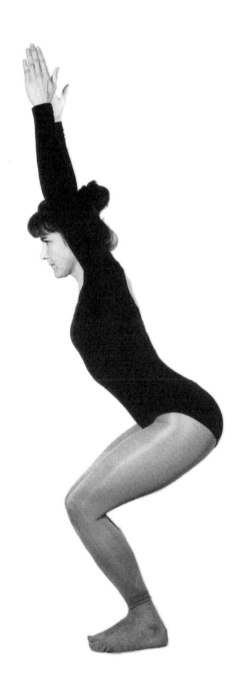

7. *Virabhadrasana* (Warrior)

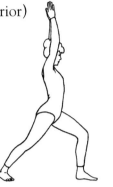

8. *Adhomukha Shvanasana* (Downward Dog)

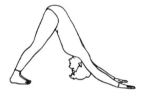

9. *Sukhasana* (Easy Pose)

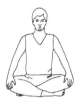

10. *Vajrasana* (Thunderbolt)

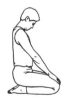

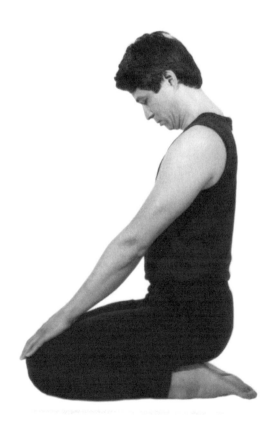

11. *Paschimatanasana* (Seated Forward Bend)

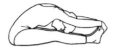

12. *Maha Mudra*

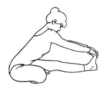

13. *Dvipada Pitham* (Desk)

14. *Urdhva Prasrita Padasana* (Leg Raises)

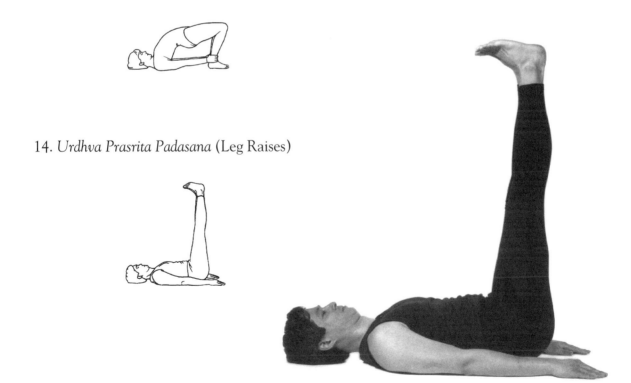

15. *Chakravakasana* (Sunbird)

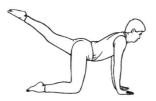

16. *Bhujangasana* (Cobra)

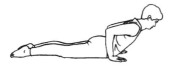

17. *Shalabhasana* (Locust)

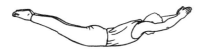

18. *Jathara Parivritti* (Lying Twist)

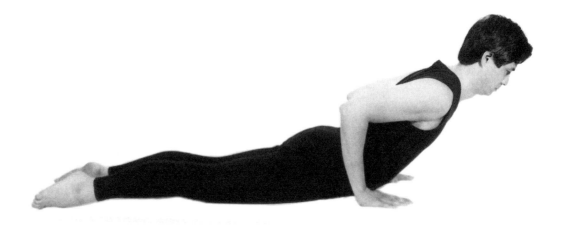

19. *Apanasana* (Knees to Chest)

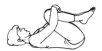

20. *Shavasana* (Relaxation Pose)

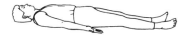

1. Samasthiti (Standing Pose)

sama - equal   *sthiti* - stay

Classically, every asana practice began with a prayer to God, Patanjali, and the student's teacher. This endowed the practice with a meaning and significance beyond its being simply a series of physical exercises. Samasthiti, often the first posture in a practice, can include *anjali mudra* (palms facing each other in prayer position), which is a symbol of that prayer.

In this asana the student can focus inside, assess him- or herself, and create the state of balance that assures a successful practice. The prayer in this posture serves as a pause. It separates the practice from one's previous physical and mental activities and brings the student's full attention to the present. In effect, it is a brief moment of intentional reintegration. It may be done when beginning a practice, or before or after each posture as the student feels appropriate, and serves as a valuable reminder of the larger aim of yoga.

Standing pose can be either a beginning of the entire practice, or the starting point for each posture. As such, it forms the basis for many others. Its Sanskrit meaning, as well as its function, deals with equality or balance. This quality is particularly critical as you begin your practice, when you establish your base (both physical and mental), which should be firm, secure, and stable. Without this balance at the beginning of your practice, it is difficult to achieve the qualities of steadiness and comfort (sthira and sukha).

We have described yoga as a progression from one point to another, higher, point. We have also said that to accomplish this movement or discovery, you must know something about your point of origin. Only then is it possible to determine how to proceed and, later, to be able to evaluate your progress by looking back for a comparison. Samasthiti should serve as a method of assessing your present state of body, mind, and breath, in order to determine what sort of practice will be most useful and appropriate to perform next.

A good teacher will use samasthiti as a posture with which to observe a student's alignment and natural posture. It is difficult to observe your own structure, even with the help of a mirror. In practicing alone, therefore, it is vitally important to become aware of your own body, so that your practice stays current and relevant to your needs. Observing your breath will help you do this.

The Classical Posture

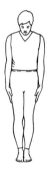

Feet are together, flat on the floor, with equal pressure on each foot.
The body is straight and balanced.
The arms are at the sides of the body.
The chin is on the chest (*jalandhara bandha*). This lowering of the head, in addition to its physical effects, brings about the proper mental state for asana. My teacher, Shri Krishnamacharya, said, "Never lose your head — keep your head down." Asana practice should not increase the ego.

The Modified Version

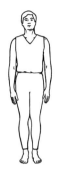

The head can be held straight. The toes may face slightly outward, with the heels together or slightly apart, whichever feels more comfortable and provides a steady, balanced base of support. This variation may make the position steadier and more comfortable.

Note: When the feet are together, the position of the pelvis changes and may cause a tightening in the back, outer hip, and leg muscles. This, in turn, disturbs your balance. A firm base of support is extremely important for the correct practice of any posture. Particularly here, as you begin your practice or posture, adjust the stance to assure steadiness and comfort (sthira and sukha).

Vinyasa Krama

Strictly speaking, standing pose involves no steps or movement. Its essence is balance and, as such, its beginning and end are the same. A useful vinyasa krama, however, is to raise your arms above your head on the inhale. Ideally, the arms end up by the ears, the palms touching and the elbows straight. Lower your arms on the exhale.

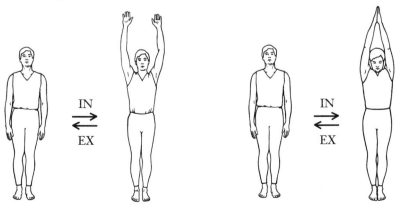

In this movement the arms may be raised either by moving forward and up, or out to the sides. Practice both variations, and notice the different effects. As always, the benefits vary according to the individual.

Modification

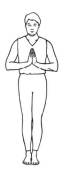

When you add anjali mudra to standing pose you can change the quality of a practice or posture. Considered one of the highest mudras, or symbols, this position initiates an attitude of prayer. The hands are placed in prayer position, palms together, with the base of the thumbs touching the chest at the base of the sternum. According to the ancient texts, this point is where God resides in the body.

One important comment on anjali mudra: The intention with which this gesture is done is its most significant aspect, and reflects the quality of a student's attitude. Mindless movement, mudras, or postures may be helpful on some levels, but do not advance a student's process of personal reintegration as quickly as when they are performed with awareness.

2. Parshva Uttanasana (Asymmetrical Forward Bend)

parshva - one side   *uttana* - to stretch

The Classical Posture

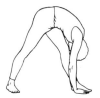

One foot is placed one pace forward.
The rear foot is turned outward 45° - 60°.
Both legs are straight.
The torso is folded over the front leg.
The hands are placed flat on the floor on each side of the front foot.
The forehead touches the leg, and the chin rests on the chest.

The Modified Version

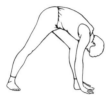

The front knee may be bent.
Fingers touch the floor.
Forehead need not touch the leg.
Chin need not be on the chest.

Vinyasa Krama

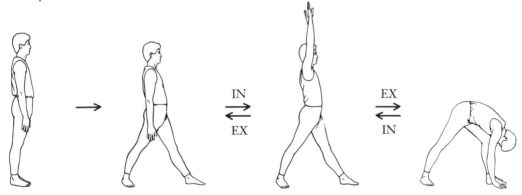

From standing pose, turn the rear foot out to 45°- 60° and take a large step forward. The distance between your feet should be one long pace; you should be able to return to standing pose in one smooth step.

Raise your arms on the inhale, from the front, with your palms facing forward at the top.

Exhale, as your torso folds forward until your palms rest lightly on the floor. Your hands should not bear any weight.

To come up, first raise your arms, then your upper back, and finally your lower back and entire torso to a vertical position. This is done on a single inhale.

Other Modifications

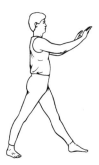

1. You may limit the arm movement, lifting your arms to a comfortable height, and bending your elbows.

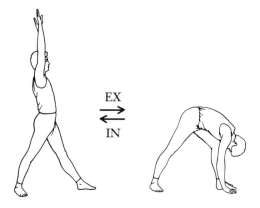

2. Bend the front leg. You can begin the movement with straight legs, bending your torso until you feel tension in the leg, then softening the knee to allow the movement of the torso to continue into the completed pose.

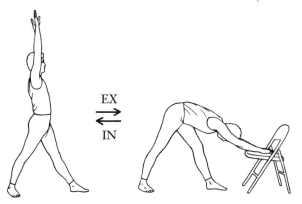

3. You may use a chair or table, so that your torso does not need to bend so far forward. Your hands will come to rest on the chair rather than the floor. Your front leg is bent.

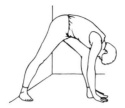

4. Place your back foot against the wall for increased stability.

These modifications also apply to most other standing postures. Bending the forward knee can be used on all standing asymmetrical postures. The way that you use these modifications will vary according to the characteristics of the student and the posture.

Notes

In the asymmetrical forward bend, as in all postures, the initial stance is extremely important, as it must provide a stable base for movement and balance. The front foot should be separated from the back by one large step. If this distance is too small it won't allow sufficient stretching; if it is too great the stance will be unsteady, balance will be difficult, and the weight will tend to shift toward the front foot. There will be little support from the back foot.

The weight should be balanced evenly between the feet, the hands bearing no weight. It is often helpful to consciously place weight on the back heel to insure stability and balance in your stance. The rear foot should be firmly on the floor. The angle of the rear foot should be between 45° - 60°.

The feet are aligned so that both heels form a line. The shoulders and upper torso face forward, with the shoulders horizontally even. One shoulder should not be higher than the other. Due to the angle of the rear foot, the hips will turn slightly. The main object is stability, rather than exactness of the angles involved, so that the emphasis is on the function rather than the form of the posture.

Asymmetrical forward bends can be useful for the observation and correction of asymmetry in the body.

Balancing Postures

Note: Balancing postures should be repeated.

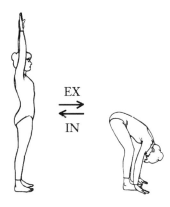

EX
IN

Uttanasana

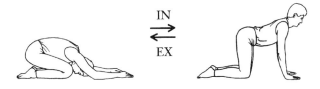

IN
EX

Chakravakasana

3. Uttanasana (Standing Forward Bend)

uttana - stretch

The Classical Posture

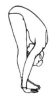

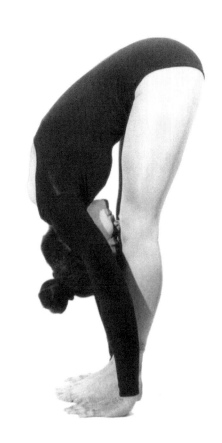

Feet are together, flat on the floor.
The legs are straight.
The torso is bent forward over the legs.
The hands are placed flat on the floor on each side of the feet.
The forehead touches the legs, and the chin is on the chest.

The Modified Version

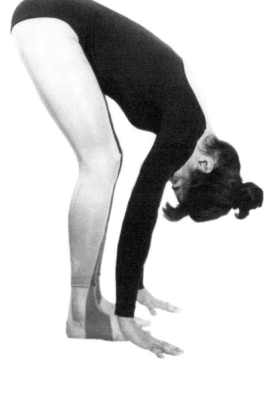

The feet may be slightly apart.
The knees are slightly bent.
The hands may touch the feet or ankles.

Vinyasa Krama

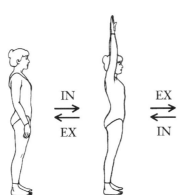 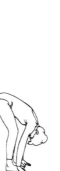

Begin in standing pose. As you breathe in, raise your arms forward and up, so that your palms face forward at the top. Bend forward on the exhale, until your hands rest on the floor.

To come up, inhale as you raise the arms first, then arch the back as the torso returns to a standing position.

Keep your head slightly down, both bending forward and returning to standing.

Other Modifications

The feet may be placed slightly apart, in a comfortable stance, in all of the following modifications. You may also return to standing with a rounded back.

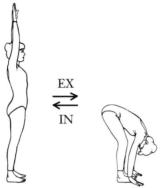

1. You may allow the knees to bend so that the torso can bend forward enough to let the hands touch the floor. To determine the right amount of bending, begin the movement with straight legs, move your torso forward until you begin to feel tension in the hamstrings, and then bend your knees.

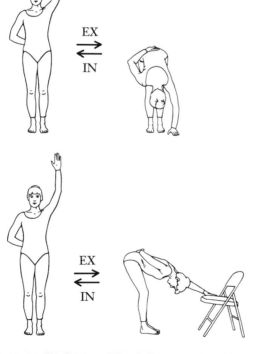

2. With one hand resting comfortably at the back or side, raise one arm and bend forward to a chair or the floor. Repeat a few times, and then change arms.

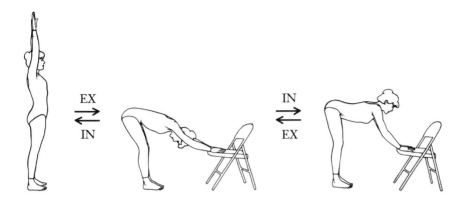

3. To use a chair, bend forward only to the point where your hands rest on the chair, but without placing weight on them. Arch your back and raise your head on the inhale. Round your back and lower your head on the exhale. Repeat this a few times. You may choose to come to the top of the chair or to the seat of the chair.

Breathing Modifications

1. You can increase the work on the back by coming out of the pose in several breaths. Arch your back and lift partially out of the pose, returning down on each exhale. With each breath lift a little higher, until you come back to standing.
2. Return to a vertical position with a long inhalation while arching the back. This will also increase the work on the back.
3. Move into the posture after exhalation, holding your breath. This will strengthen your abdomen.
4. You can use uttanasana as a warm-up pose by adjusting the breath and movement, so that the inhale and exhale are both about four seconds long. Repeat this several times.

Variations of Uttanasana

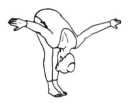

1. Spread your arms out to the side.

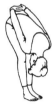

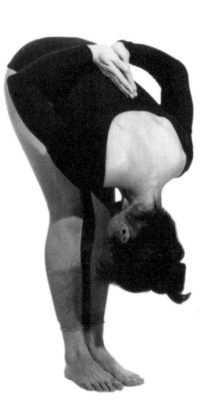

2. Cross your hands behind the back, fingers interlocked.

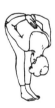

3. Bring your palms together behind your back.

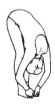

4. Hold on to your big toes (*padangusthasana*).

5. Place the palms of your hands under the soles of the feet (*padahastasana*).

Balancing Postures

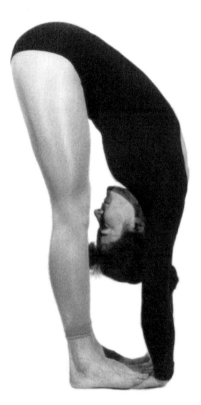

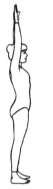 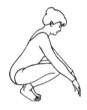

Squat

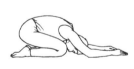 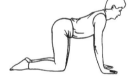

Chakravakasana

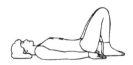 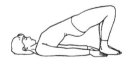

Dvipada pitham

4. Ardha Uttanasana (Half Forward Bend)

ardha - half   *uttana* - to stretch

The Classical Posture

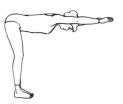

Feet are together, flat on the floor.

The legs are completely straight. The torso is bent forward at a near right angle to the legs.

The back is arched.

The arms are extended overhead.

The chin is on the chest.

The Modified Version

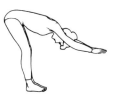

The feet may be slightly apart, in a comfortably stable position.

The knees and arms may be slightly bent.

Vinyasa Krama

Each vinyasa below has a different effect.

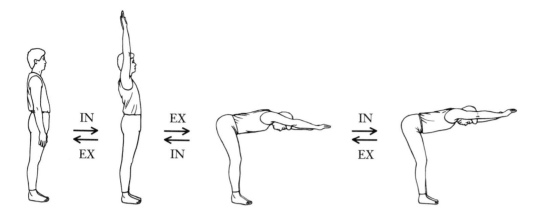

1. Begin standing. Exhale into a half forward bend. Breathe in, extend your back and arms, and exhale in place. Inhale back up to standing.

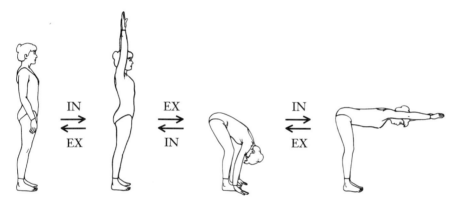

2. Begin standing. Inhale and raise your arms forward and up, and exhale into uttanasana. Inhale halfway up, arching your back and extending your arms. Exhale down. Inhale up to standing.

Balancing Postures

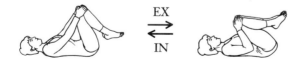

Apanasana

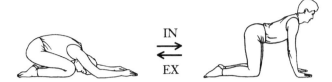

Chakravakasana

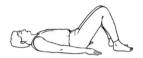

Rest with knees bent

5. Ardha Utkatasana (Chair)

ardha - half   *utkata* - squat

The Classical Posture

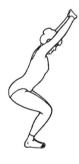

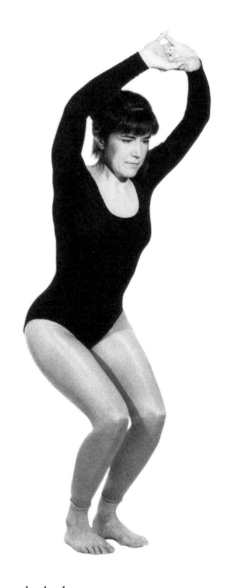

Feet are together, flat on the floor.
Knees are bent and held together.
Back is arched.
Arms are raised above head, close to ears, with the fingers interlocked, palms turned upward.
Chin is on the chest.

The Modified Version

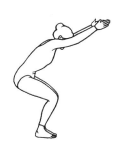

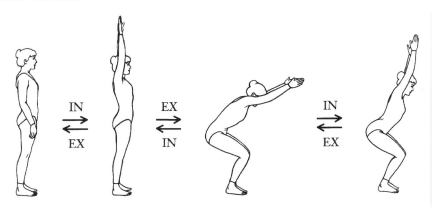

Feet may be spread to a comfortable position.
Arms may be bent, palms facing forward, keeping
the shoulders lowered and relaxed.

Vinyasa Krama

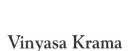

Begin in standing pose. Inhale and raise your arms forward and up.
Exhale into half squat position with a slightly rounded back. Inhale and arch
into position.

Balancing Postures

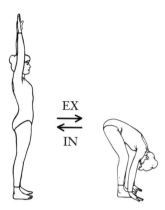

Uttanasana, repeated

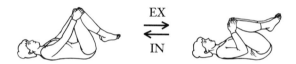

Apanasana

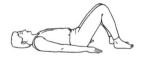

Rest with bent knees

6. Utthita Trikonasana (Triangle)

utthita - standing   *trikona* - triangle

We will present two forms of utthita trikonasana: the standing twist and the lateral bend. These two positions have quite different effects and levels of difficulty. The strength and condition of the student's torso will determine which is the more appropriate asana to select. The lateral bend should always be performed with a degree of caution.

1. *Utthita Trikonasana to the Opposite Side: Standing Twist*

The Classical Posture

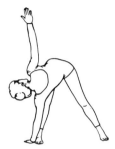

Feet are spread one step apart to a position that allows one to return smoothly to samasthiti, and to stand comfortably and firmly.

Feet are parallel and legs are straight.

The torso is parallel to the floor, twisted so that the opposite shoulder is closest to the floor.

Arms are extended sideways at shoulder level, with one hand lightly on the floor at the outside of the foot, but not bearing any weight.

The head remains in line with the spine and is turned to face upward toward the upper hand.

The Modified Version

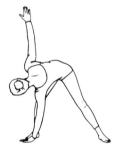

Feet may turn out slightly. The leg toward which you turn may be bent. The head may be left in line with the torso, rather than twisting it upwards.

Vinyasa Krama

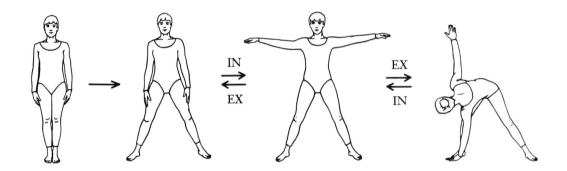

Begin by first bending the torso slightly forward before twisting. The body is more accustomed to bending forward than to twisting; this slight adaptation will make the posture easier. Let the knee toward which you are moving bend enough to release your torso to the side.

As you stay and breathe in the posture, you will feel the twist in the abdomen by gently moving deeper into the twist with each exhale.

To return, twist up as you move toward the center. If you move to the center and then twist up, the action is more of a forward bend than a twist. Inhale as you return to center.

2. Utthita Trikonasana to the Same Side: Lateral Bend

This posture is the more difficult of the two, and should be practiced with caution, particularly when holding the pose.

The Classical Posture

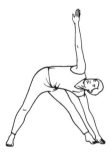

Standing position is the same as for above.

Torso is parallel to the floor, facing forward and aligned directly over the leg.

Arms are extended out from shoulders in a vertical line from the floor upward, the hand at the outside of the foot touching the floor without bearing weight.

Head faces upward toward the top hand, in line with the spine.

The Modified Version

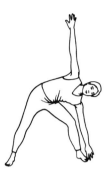

The body need not be in line with the legs.
The head need not be turned towards the upper hand.
The knees can be slightly bent.

Vinyasa Krama

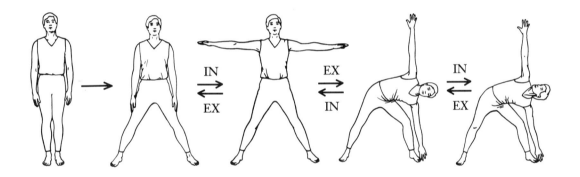

On the exhale, begin by bending the torso slightly forward before lateral bending. Let the knee toward which you are moving bend enough to release your torso to the side. On the inhale, straighten your torso, bringing it parallel to the floor.

Balancing Postures for Standing Twist and Lateral Bend

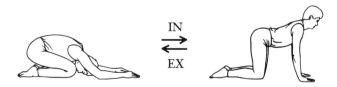

Chakravakasana

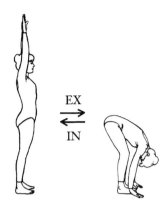

Uttanasana

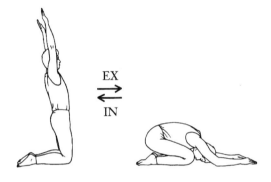

Vajrasana

Paschimatanasana

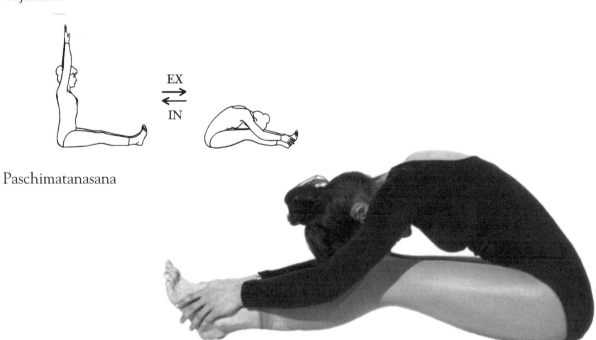

7. Virabhadrasana (Warrior)

Virabhadra - one of Shiva's warriors

The Classical Posture

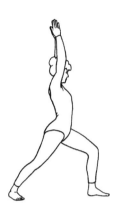

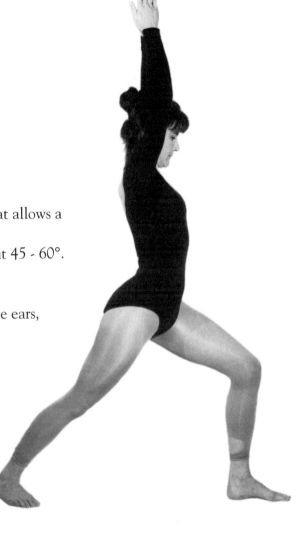

One leg is forward, at a maximum distance that allows a return without strain.

The back leg is straight. Turn the back foot out 45 - 60°.

The back is arched, but remains vertical.

The head faces forward.

Arms are straight, raised above the head by the ears, with the palms together.

The Modified Version

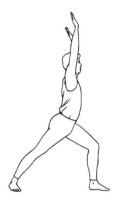

You may bend your arms.

The head may be slightly raised.

Vinyasa Krama

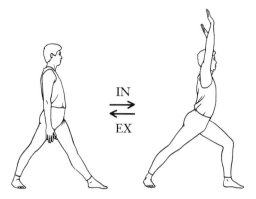

Begin in a wide stance, with your back foot turned out, both legs straight, and your arms at your sides. As you inhale, bend your front knee, raise your arms forward and up, gently arching your back.

Other Modifications

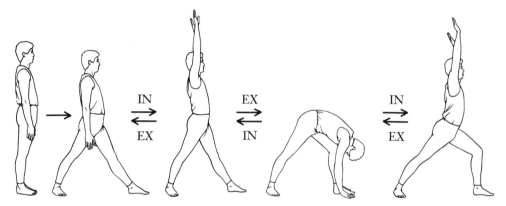

Move into asymmetrical forward bend. As you come out of the pose, inhale, raising your arms and arching your back. Repeat on the other side.

Notes

Both legs must be active in the posture; if the back leg is inactive, the work goes to the thigh rather than to the back. Also, if the angle of the bent leg is not proper, the weight will be transferred into the thigh, away from the back.

Balancing Postures

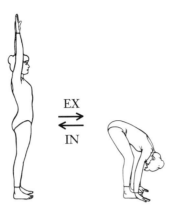

Uttanasana

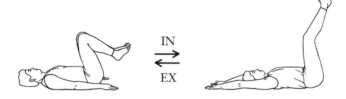

Leg Raises

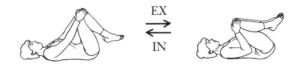

Apanasana

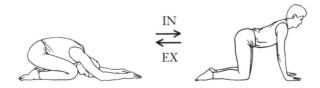

Chakravakasana

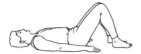

Rest with knees bent

8. Adhomukha Shvanasana (Downward Dog)

adho - down   *mukha* - face   *shvana* - dog

The Classical Posture

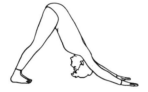

Toes and hands are on the floor, with the heels as close to the floor as possible.

Legs are straight.

The weight of the upper body is evenly distributed on the hands and feet.

The chin is on the chest, and the top of the head is on the floor.

The Modified Version

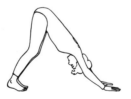

Heels can come off the floor.

Feet may be separated, about hips' distance apart.

Knees may be bent.

The arms do not have to be rigid or straight.

The head is off the floor, in line with the spine.

The chin does not come to chest.

Vinyasa Krama

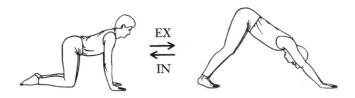

Begin from chakravakasana. On the exhale, move into the downward dog pose. Reverse the sequence and repeat.

Note: Refer to page 39 for additional vinyasas.

Notes

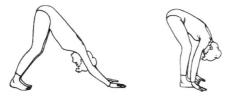

In downward dog pose the weight is on the shoulders. Because of this and because of the angle of the shoulders, this pose will increase neck tension. Contrast this with uttanasana (standing forward bend), where you still get the inversion effect, but without the strain on the shoulders. Downward dog can be used for the practice of the bandhas (see Chapter 6).

Balancing Postures

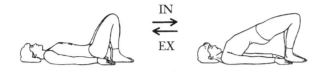

Dvipada pitham

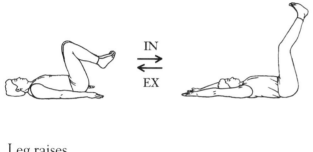

Leg raises

9. Sukhasana (Easy Pose)

sukham - comfortable

The Classical Posture

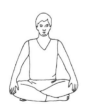

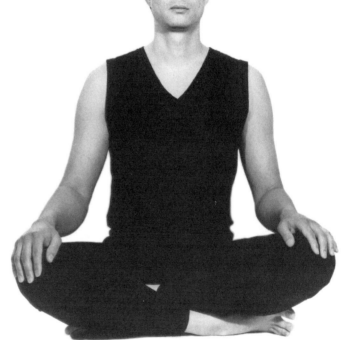

The torso is straight in the seated position.
The spine must be held erect to enable proper breathing.
Legs are bent and crossed, with each foot under the opposite knee.
The chin is on the chest.
The arms are straight, palms on the knees.

The Modified Version

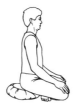

A pillow may be used, lifting the hips off the floor.
Arms can be relaxed, with hands resting comfortably on the thighs.
Head is erect.

Vinyasa Krama

Sit on the floor. Cross your legs, with each foot under the opposite knee. Place your palms on your knees.

Notes

Sukhasana is one of the basic positions for pranayama practice. The two prerequisites are that the student be comfortable sitting on the floor, and able to easily hold the spine erect.

There should be no ill effects from a posture after it is completed. Sukhasana is a static pose, so there is a greater chance of pain in the knees, ankles, or back after a lengthy stay in it. You must prepare adequately and correctly for prolonged periods in this posture.

Sukhasana provides stability for sitting, and allows you to maintain a straight spine, which is necessary for pranayama practice. This posture is only effective if it is steady and comfortable. Although pranayama seated on the floor provides a different feeling from sitting in a chair, without ease and steadiness it is not suitable.

Related Postures

There are several other postures used for pranayama or reflection. In each, the configuration of the spine is slightly different. It is very important to choose the correct posture, because an uncomfortable posture may cause pain and associated problems in other areas when done for a lengthy period.

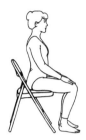

1. Sit in a chair with your spine erect and feet on the floor.

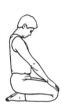 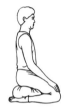

2. In vajrasana, the spine is easily held erect, as the heels act as a pillow. Still, some people will feel pain in the ankles or knees. You may also use a support in this posture.

Balancing Posture

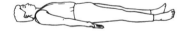

Shavasana

10. Vajrasana (Thunderbolt)

vajra - thunderbolt

The Classical Posture

Kneeling on the floor with legs together.
Sitting on the heels, keeping the torso straight.
Arms are straight with the palms on the knees.
Chin is on the chest.

The Modified Version

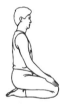

Elbows can be bent, palms resting on the knees
or thighs.
Head is straight.

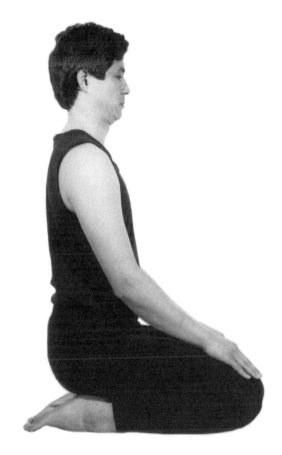

Vinyasa Krama

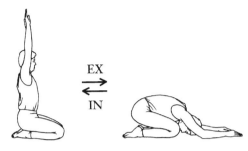

1. Sitting on your heels, raise your arms on the inhale and bend forward on the exhale.

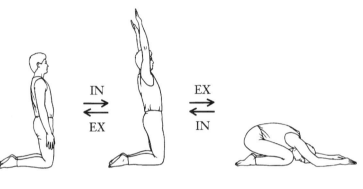

2. From a kneeling position, raise your arms on the inhale. Bend forward on the exhale.

Balancing Posture

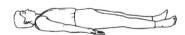

Shavasana

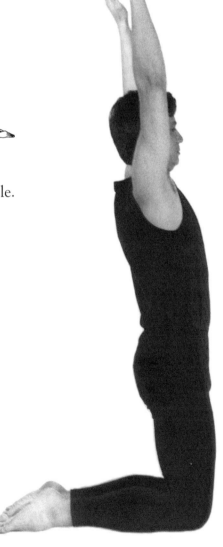

11. Paschimatanasana (Seated Forward Bend)

paschima - lower back   *tana* - stretch

The Classical Posture

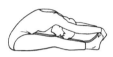

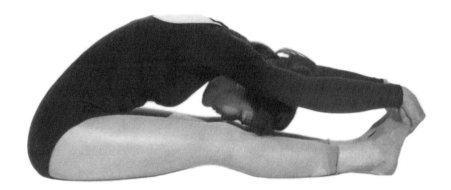

Seated on the floor, legs are together and straight, feet vertical.

The torso is folded over the legs.

The arms are slightly bent, extended above the head, hands holding the feet from the sides and fingers folding over arches.

The forehead is on the legs.

The chin is on the chest.

The Modified Version

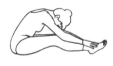

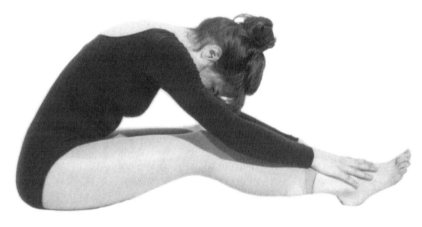

The knees may be bent. To determine the proper amount of bending, start from sitting upright, and begin bending forward until you feel some resistance in your legs. Then bend your knees enough to allow for work in the back. Keep this knee position as you move in and out of the posture, so that you can focus on your back.

Hands may be positioned comfortably on the legs or knees.

Feet may be separated slightly.

The forehead need not come all the way down to the legs.

The head is in a neutral position.

Vinyasa Krama

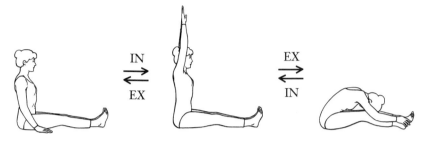

Sit on the floor with your legs straight. Inhaling, raise your arms overhead from the front. Exhaling, fold your torso over your legs, so that your forehead touches your legs, and your hands are holding your feet. Inhale, coming up with your back arched.

Note: When staying in the posture, use your breath to deepen the pose, releasing further into it on the exhale. If you use your arms to pull your torso down, you will produce tension in your shoulders and neck.

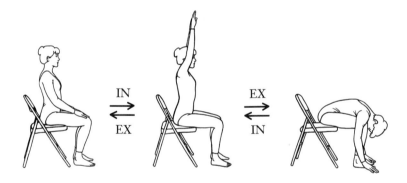

This posture may also be done using a chair. This lessens the stretch on your legs enough to release your lower back into a position that stretches it.

Other Modifications

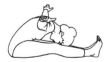

1.   Your arms may be spread out to your sides.

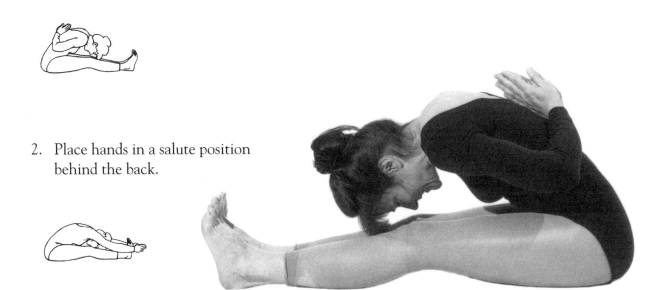

2. Place hands in a salute position behind the back.

3. Extend your hands beyond your feet, with your palms together.

Balancing Postures

This posture is often done at the end of a practice, and serves as a balance posture in itself. However, if it is done intensely and/or is difficult for a student, the following postures are suitable to balance it.

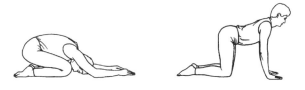

Chakravakasana

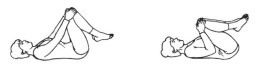

Apanasana

12. Maha Mudra

maha - great   *mudra* - symbol

The Classical Posture

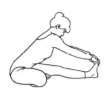

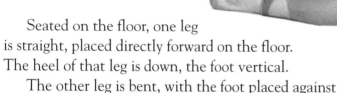

Seated on the floor, one leg
is straight, placed directly forward on the floor.
The heel of that leg is down, the foot vertical.
The other leg is bent, with the foot placed against
the inner thigh (groin) of the straight leg, as near to the body as possible.
The straight leg forms a right angle with hips.
Shoulders are level horizontally, and face squarely forward.
The chin is on the chest and the arms are straight.
The torso is folded forward from the waist, so that the fingers can hold
the sole of the foot.
The back is straight.
Arms are straight, the hands holding the soles of the feet.
All three bandhas are practiced in this posture. (See Chapter 6.)

The Modified Version

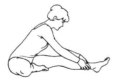

The hands may hold shin, knee, or ankle.
The knee may be slightly bent.
The elbows may be bent to reduce tension in the shoulders.
The chin moves down toward the chest.
The posture can be done without the bandhas.

Vinyasa Krama

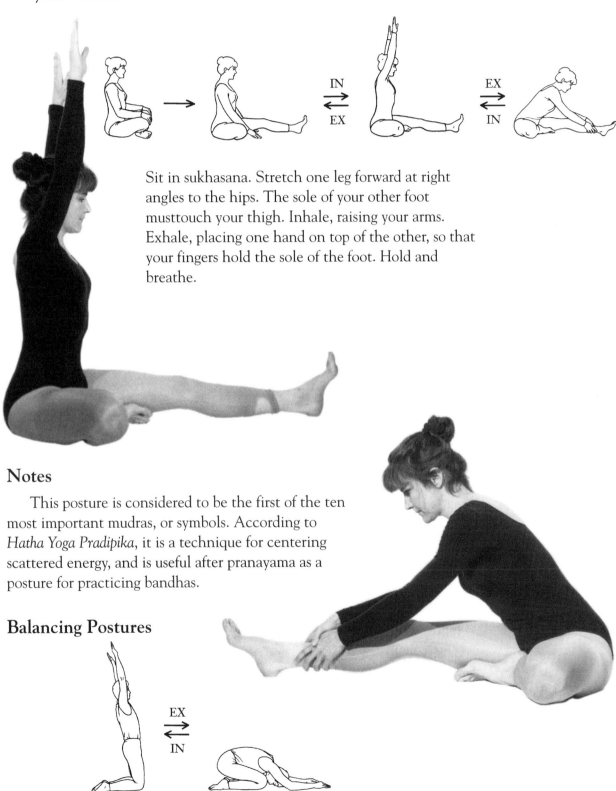

Sit in sukhasana. Stretch one leg forward at right angles to the hips. The sole of your other foot musttouch your thigh. Inhale, raising your arms. Exhale, placing one hand on top of the other, so that your fingers hold the sole of the foot. Hold and breathe.

Notes

This posture is considered to be the first of the ten most important mudras, or symbols. According to *Hatha Yoga Pradipika*, it is a technique for centering scattered energy, and is useful after pranayama as a posture for practicing bandhas.

Balancing Postures

Vajrasana

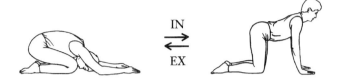

Chakravakasana

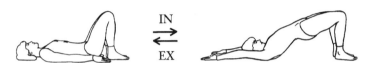

Dvipada pitham

13. Dvipada Pitham (Desk)

dvi - two   *pada* - feet   *pitham* - desk

The Classical Posture

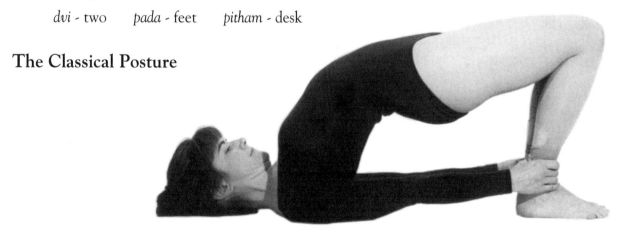

The torso and legs are raised off the floor and supported by the head, shoulders, and feet.

The head is on the floor, and the chin is on the chest.

The feet are together, flat on the floor, with the lower legs almost vertical.

Knees are together.

The hands are holding the ankles.

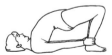

The Modified Version

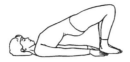

The knees may be separated.
Feet are apart in a parallel stance.
Arms are straight, with palms down on the floor.
The head rests on the floor in a neutral position.

Vinyasa Krama

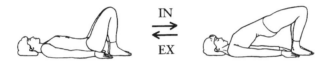

On the inhale, press your feet into the floor, and then lift your torso.
On the exhale, if necessary for stability, press your hands slightly, and then lower your torso.

Modification

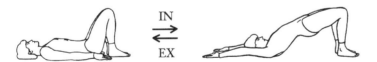

You may raise your arms overhead as your torso lifts on the inhale.

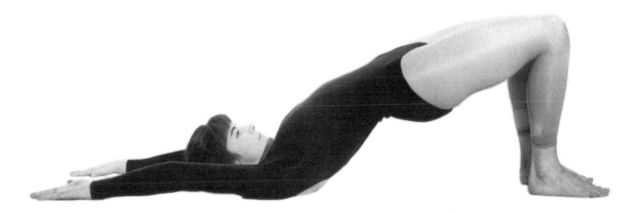

Notes

It is important to keep the head fixed during movement, in order to alleviate stress on your neck and allow the work to remain in your upper back. This takes some attention, since the head naturally tends to move backward during the lift.

Balancing Posture

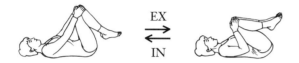

Apanasana

14. Urdhva Prasrita Padasana (Leg Raises)

urdhva - upward   *prasrita* - extended   *pada* - legs

The Classical Posture

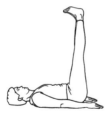

Lying on the back with the head on the floor.
Chin is on the chest.
Legs are together and straight, at right angles to the floor.
Arms are straight on the floor by your side.

Vinyasa Krama

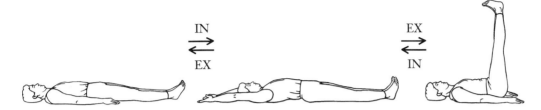

Lying on the back, raise the arms overhead on the inhale. Lower your arms as you raise the legs on the exhale. Your raised legs stay at right angles to the floor.

Modifications

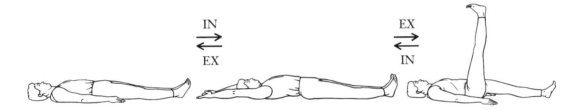

1. Raise one leg on exhale.

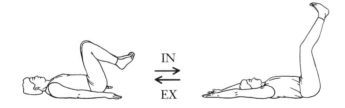

2. From apanasana, raise your arms and legs on the inhale. Your legs may be bent.

Balancing Postures

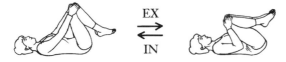

Apanasana

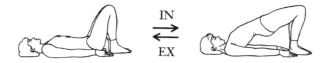

Dvipada pitham

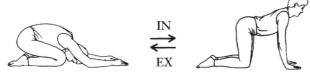

Chakravakasana

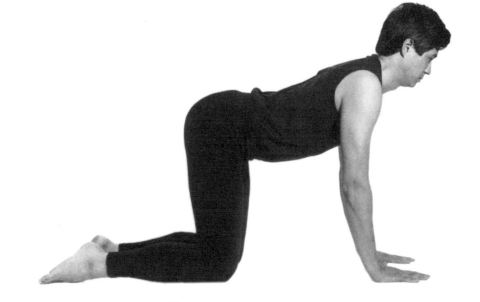

15. Chakravakasana (Sunbird)

chakravaka - mythological bird

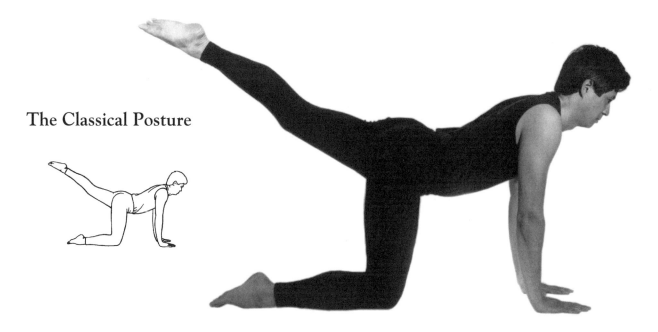

The Classical Posture

Kneeling on the floor, one straight leg is raised higher than the hip.
The back is arched.
The head is raised to face forward.
The elbows are straight, with the palms flat on floor supporting the torso.
The hands are placed at shoulders' width, fingers and thumbs together, hands parallel.

The Modified Version

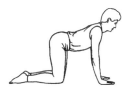

The leg is not lifted; only the back moves into the arch.
Knees may separated to a comfortable distance (about hips' width apart).
The head is lifted only slightly.

Vinyasa Krama

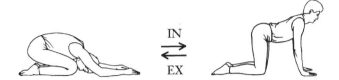

On the inhale, gently arch your back and look forward. As you exhale, sit back on your heels, lowering your torso, head, and arms to the floor.

Modification

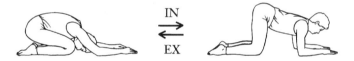

Rest on your elbows rather than on your hands.

Balancing Posture

This posture is often considered to be a balance posture itself, and therefore needs no other, except shavasana.

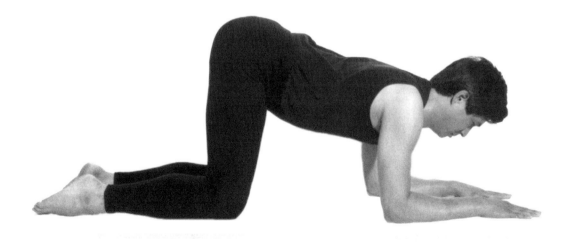

16. Bhujangasana (Cobra)

bhujangam - snake

The Classical Pose

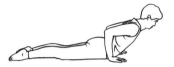

Lying down on the stomach, it is started at the navel, raising the chest, shoulders, and head off the floor.

The head is in line with the spine, facing forward.

The hands are flat on the floor at navel level, close to the body.

Elbows are bent and held close to the body.

The hands should only slightly support the torso, not pressing hard into the floor.

The legs are straight together.

The Modified Version

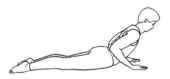

The legs may be separated.

The hands may be moved up toward the shoulders and slightly away from the body to support the back. This transfers the effort away from the back toward the shoulders themselves. In some cases, work is needed more in one area than the other, so adjusting your arm position can not only facilitate the purpose of the asana, but also provide a safety measure.

Vinyasa Krama

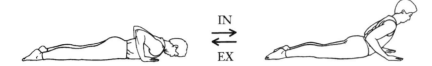

The torso lifts on the inhale and lowers on the exhale.

Notes

When staying in the posture, the body will naturally lift on each inhale, and slightly lower on the exhale. Keeping this drop to a minimum results in significant strengthening of the back and torso.

Your natural tendency in this posture will be to lift your head, because it feels as though this arches your spine. In fact, it simply compresses the vertebrae in the neck area. Instead, keep your head in its normal relationship to the spine.

Modification

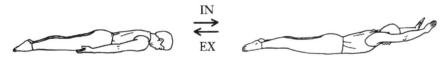

Begin with your arms at your side. On the inhale, sweep arms forward as you lift your torso.

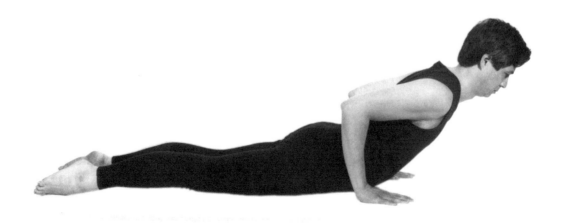

Balancing Postures

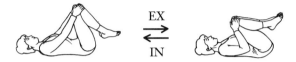

Apanasana

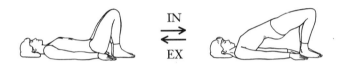

Dvipada pitham

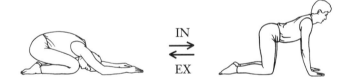

Chakravakasana

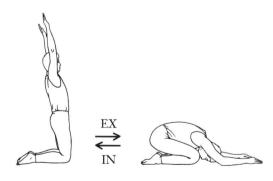

Vajrasana

17. Shalabhasana (Locust)

shalabha - locust

The Classical Posture

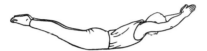

Lying down on the stomach with forehead to the floor.

The chest, shoulders, head, and legs are raised.

The arms are extended above the head close to the ears with palms held together.

The legs are straight and held together.

Note: Lifting the legs alone is not advised, because chest pressure is increased, thereby also increasing your heart rate, and heightening tension in the cervical spine.

The Modified Version

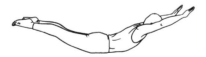

The legs may be spread apart.

Knees may be bent.

Arms are extended without bringing the palms together.

The arms may be bent.

Vinyasa Krama

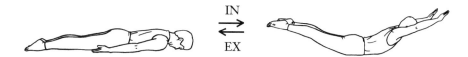

1. Lie on your stomach with your forehead to the floor. Your arms are by your sides, with your legs straight and together. Inhale, raising your legs first, followed by your chest, head and arms. Sweep your arms to the front, and extend them above your head. Exhaling, return to a prone position.

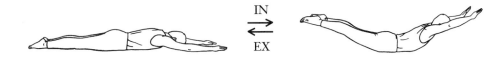

2. Starting with your arms above your head on the floor is more difficult than sweeping them up from the sides.

Other Modifications

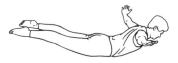

1. Your arms may be spread out to the sides.

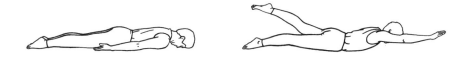

2. *Ardha Shalabhasana* (asymmetrical locust). Lift one leg and one arm at a time. This can be done lifting the arm and leg on the same side of the body, or on opposite sides. When lifting one leg, keep the hip on that side on the ground to prevent rolling.

Balancing Postures

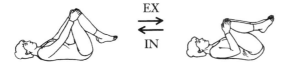

Apanasana

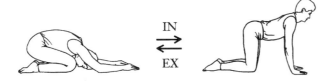

Chakravakasana

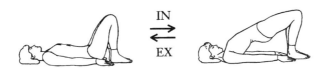

Dvipada pitham

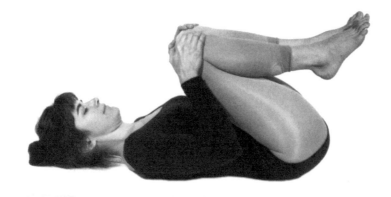

18. Jathara Parivritti (Lying Twist)

jathara - abdominal   *pari* - other than
vritti - movement (other than normal movement of the abdominals)

The Classical Posture

Lying on the back, the legs are straight and held together on the floor, forming an acute angle with body.

The arms are extended on the floor at right angles to the torso.

The hand on the same side as the feet holds the top foot with the entire hand.

The head is turned away from the feet.

The Modified Version

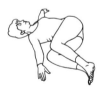

The feet may be not held at all.

The head may remain in the center.

The arms may be relaxed and placed lower than shoulder level.

The legs may be bent.

Note: This posture requires considerable effort in the neck and should not be done by students with neck problems.

Vinyasa Krama

There are several steps to reach the final position. The correct use of the breath is very important.

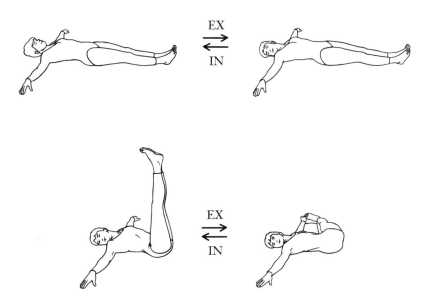

Inhale as your arms move to the side, not touching the floor as they move.

Exhaling, lift your head, turn it to the side, and release it to floor, with your ear on the ground. Be sure that this is a lifting motion, and not a rolling one, as the latter will leave the head misaligned over the spine.

Inhale in place.

Exhale, and raise your legs to a right angle with the torso. As your legs lower to one side, grab the big toes with your hand.

Using the exhale when raising your legs helps decrease the abdominal resistance to lifting this large amount of weight.

(You may stay in this position 6 - 8 breaths before returning.)

To return, inhale and lift your legs up to center.

Exhale in place.

Inhale, and lower your legs to your starting position on the floor.

Return your head to center — or, you can return by lifting your legs up to center and down to the floor on one inhale. Then return your head to center.

Other Modifications

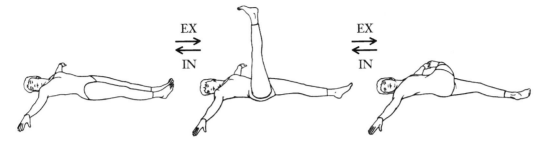

1. Raise only one leg, crossing over the straight leg to the opposite side.

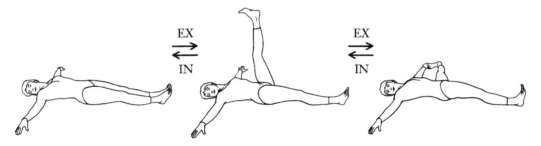

2. Raise one leg, then lower it to same side, holding it with your hand on the same side of your body.

Balancing Postures

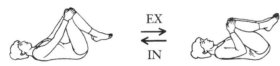

Apanasana

Rest with knees bent

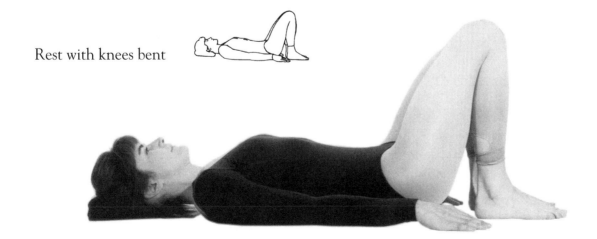

19. Apanasana (Knees to Chest)

apana - lower abdomen

The Classical Posture

Lying on the back, the head is on the floor.
The legs are together with knees bent, folded into the chest.
The hips and buttocks are on the floor.
Elbows are bent, with the hands clasped around the knees.
The chin is on the chest.

The Modified Version

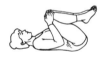

The legs can be spread a comfortable distance apart.
The hands can hold either the outsides or the tops of the knees.
The arms may be relaxed, creating no tension in shoulders.
The legs may fold down just to a comfortable position.
The head rests on the floor in a neutral position.

Vinyasa Krama

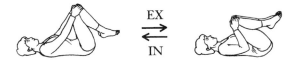

On the exhale, fold your knees gently toward your chest. Your arms should guide with only minimal pressure and effort. On the inhale, release the pressure and allow your legs to move slightly away from your body.

Notes

The lower abdomen is considered by Ayurveda to contain impurities. It is seen as the seat of disease in the body. Apanasana works this area, removing blockages due to impurities, and thus restoring the smooth flow of exhalation. Exhalation is thought to be responsible for the elimination of these impurities.

Balancing Posture

This posture is generally used as a balancing posture and requires no other except shavasana.

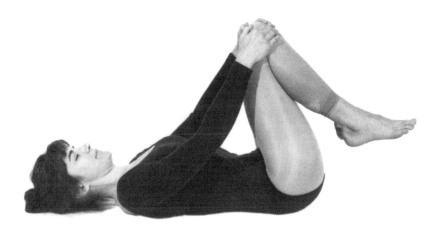

20. Shavasana (Relaxation Pose)

shava - corpse

The Classical Posture

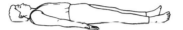

Lying on the back, the body is straight, but relaxed.
Feet are slightly apart.
The arms are near the sides, slightly away from body, palms up or down.
The position should feel absolutely comfortable.

The Modified Version

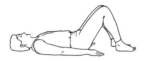

The knees may be bent, the feet on the floor.

Notes

This posture is a link to relaxation, either at the end of an entire practice or as a rest or balancing position between postures. It is the posture for mental relaxation — as difficult an activity for many people as the postures themselves. Breathing should be relaxed and natural, unless some specified pranayama is intended.

A rest between postures doesn't always need to be shavasana. One may also sit on a chair, or relax in another comfortable position.

4
VIPARITA KARANI — INVERSION

The Philosophy of Inversion

Although primarily understood as "inversion," viparita karani's literal translation of "opposite process" reveals that its significance is far greater than just the idea of being physically upside down. True yoga is about continual change accomplished in an integrated manner, which means that it must involve all aspects of our being. The concept of viparita karani applies to all such aspects, helping us to change both physical and mental habits in the process.

As humans we are all conditioned by our past. We tend to operate in the present using the behavior patterns and reactions developed from earlier experiences. For most of us, these patterns are deeply ingrained and automatic, even though life around us changes constantly.

According to the *Yoga Sutras*, both habit and change are always present in life, as is the dynamic interaction between the two. Our old habits can create resistance to change and keep us stuck in the same place. Likewise, our ability to adapt to change can produce real transformation and growth. The goal of yoga practice is to bring about this kind of positive change, so that we can move from bondage to freedom. The ability to confront change *is* yoga.

Viparita karani is one way of doing this. Philosophically, this "opposite process" means looking at things from a different perspective. When we turn the body upside down, we literally see the world in a new way. Because the body and mind are deeply connected, changing one aspect affects the whole being. It is for this reason that the headstand has come to symbolize yoga.

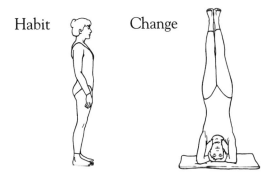

Yet viparita karani can also be any of the following postures, as each of them also involves some form of inversion:

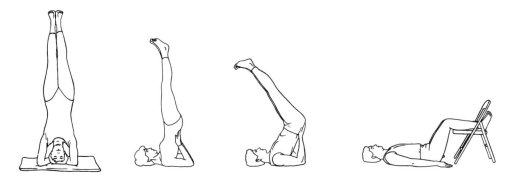

The Psychology of Inversion

Viparita karani affects your physical and psychological state. First of all, inversion is a radical change in the body's normal state. For example, its base of support is different, it changes your visual sense, movement or flight are not easily possible, and so on. You may experience emotional reactions such as fear, excitement, or addiction to the pose. These reactions can help to reveal various psychological states and to change them.

Typically the way someone reacts to the thought of doing the posture, to actually doing it, and then to bringing it to a close, demonstrates his or her willingness to take risks and to deal with changes in life. A student's ability to follow instructions in an upside-down position can indicate his or her ease in new situations. Confusion, fear, or anger may surface, as may determination or composure. After doing the posture a student's reactions will indicate not only the intensity of its effects, but also how well the student deals with those effects.

Quite often the practice of viparita karani will cause changes in one's psychology — particularly in dealing with any fears associated with the pose. If you can conquer fear on the physical level you may be better able to do so in other realms of your life. This is an important factor in learning to confront change, and is a real step toward reintegration.

A good teacher will respect a student's response — particularly if it is one of fear — and will create a gradual sequence of appropriate steps for accomplishing the pose. In some cases it may be better for the student to do another posture altogether. Strictly speaking, viparita karani merely involves elevating the feet above the head, so placing the feet on a chair serves the purpose quite well for people who are fearful, older, injured, or fatigued.

The Concept of Inversion

Viparita karani is one of the ten important mudras, according to *Hatha Yoga Pradipika*, an ancient yoga text. Mudra means "seal," and is a means of sealing certain areas of the body to enhance the removal of impurities. According to yoga and to Ayurveda, an ancient Indian system of health, impurities lie in the lower abdomen. Above this area lies the *agni*, or fire, which burns the impurities when they move near it.

In a normal upright position gravity pulls impurities and the abdomen itself downward. For this reason this area is considered the seat of sickness. When the feet are elevated above the head, this process is reversed and gravity automatically moves the dirt downward toward the fire. Correct breathing is instrumental in this reversal process, because it can burn the impurities and remove them from the body more effectively. Therefore, the ability to perform correct deep breathing is critical in inverted postures. (This will be discussed in greater detail in the chapter on pranayama.)

Another benefit of inversion is that raising the feet above the head can relieve tendencies of the blood to pool in one's legs, and can thereby improve one's general circulation. You can accomplish this simply by lifting the legs in the air, or by placing them up on a chair while lying down.

The headstand has the reputation of being a panacea, and is thought of by some as the main prerequisite to good health for anyone of any age or condition. Realistically, however, its effects vary greatly according to the individual. For students who can comfortably maintain the posture while using slow, deep breathing, it definitely brings a sense of well-being. For others, the structural effects of the pose may be harmful. For example, pregnant women and people with low or high blood pressure, neck pain, or neck injuries should avoid these postures, as they may cause discomfort and even unpleasant effects. In any case, the practice of headstand must always include proper preparation and balancing postures.

Practical Aspects of Inversion

Headstand (*salamba shirshasana*) and shoulderstand (*salamba sarvangasana*) or half-shoulderstand (viparita karani) are often linked in practice to balance each other. This discussion will focus on both postures and on the relationship between them. Because it is not wise to embark on an inversion without the advice and guidance of a good teacher, we will discuss this from the perspective of the teacher-student interaction.

The practice of inverted postures requires the following foundation:

1. Knowledge of a student's psychological and structural state.
2. Proper preparation and sequencing.
3. Appropriate adaptation.

To elaborate on these:

1. Knowledge of a student's psychological and structural state. Before recommending an inversion for a student, a teacher needs to know about the student's structure, limitations, injuries, and pains. This information will determine the state of readiness to do or learn an inverted posture. It will also provide guidelines about how the posture should be taught to that particular student.

A good teacher will observe a student standing upright, and note any structural factors or asymmetries in both the vertical and lateral axes. These factors will still be present when the person is upside down, but the shift in the directional pull of gravity will change which areas bear weight, withstand pressure, or are involved in balance. Most parts of the body will need to perform a different function when subjected to these different conditions.

2. Proper preparation and sequencing. Given the knowledge of a person's structural, functional and psychological status, a teacher will need to determine the appropriate sequence of preparation and balancing. You cannot simply jump into a posture without preparation. This is particularly true for deep backbends, postures that involve holding the breath, and inversions. An inverted posture should never be the first posture in a practice, even though it may be the main goal.

Before attempting any inversion it is necessary to have:

- A strong and healthy neck.
- The ability to breathe in an inverted position.
- A healthy muscular system, especially in one's back.

A good teacher will observe a student in some preparatory postures to determine his or her readiness. For example, observing a standing forward bend will reveal a great deal about the strength and flexibility of the person's body, including his or her back. It will also prepare the student for breathing with his or her head down, as well as demonstrating his or her ability to do this. A standing twist shows the condition of the neck. (More details and examples of sequences for shoulderstand, viparita karani, and headstand are included later in this chapter.)

The base of support must be symmetrical in inverted postures, just as it must be when standing. In the vinyasa kramas for headstand, shoulderstand, and viparita karani, the first step is to check the alignment of the body before elevating the legs.

3. Appropriate adaptation. A teacher will adapt the posture once he or she knows the student's structural limitations. For instance, a swayed back (lordosis) is still a swayed back when one is upside down, so adaptations for that condition must be included in the posture. The shape of one's head is also extremely relevant in determining how the head should be placed to provide a stable base (to be discussed later in this chapter). Likewise, the muscular development of one's shoulder girdle will have an effect on the position of the arms and elbows.

To illustrate this discussion, we will review three inversions, each in its classical form, a modification, and according to vinyasa krama.

1. Viparita Karani (Half Shoulderstand)

viparita - opposite   *karani* - process

The Classical Posture

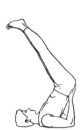

Head and shoulders are on the floor, facing upward.
The torso is straight, at about 70° to floor.
Upper arms and elbows are on the floor, parallel to each other.
The hands support the torso from the back.
Legs are straight, feet together above the head.
The legs should be positioned in such a way that there is no tension in the abdomen. Legs should be tilted toward the head, rather than toward the back, because the latter produces strain in the abdomen and neck.
Breathing should be comfortable.

The Modified Version

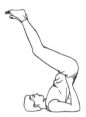

Legs may bend on the way up into the posture.
Legs may spread slightly apart to release the back.
Knees may bend slightly.
Toes and feet may relax to make breathing easier.

Vinyasa Krama

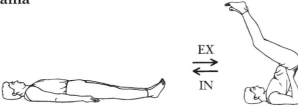

EX
IN

Begin lying on the floor, with your arms by your sides, and your legs together. First lift your head slightly, to check that your body is correctly aligned, then return your head to the floor.

On the exhale, lift your legs toward your head and allow the torso to lift off the ground as this happens. Go as far as is easily possible with just your legs, and then bring your hands to your lower back above your buttocks to support your torso.

While returning on inhale, slightly bend your knees and gently lower your torso to the floor, without lifting your head from the floor. Stay for a few breaths.

Notes

It is very important in viparita karani to be able breathe easily, slowly, and deeply. Therefore, the chin is not locked and the head should be free to move to insure this ease of breathing. Concentrate on the exhale, lengthening it as much as is comfortable. The natural effect of inversion is a shortening of the breath.

There will be weight on your wrists and elbows, which relieves the neck from supporting the majority of the body weight. The more pressure exerted in pushing the torso toward the vertical position (as in full shoulderstand), the more weight is transferred to the neck.

Balancing Postures

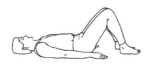

Rest with knees bent

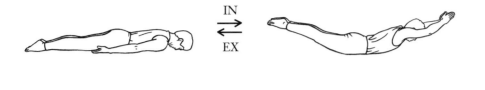

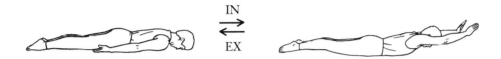

Shalabhasana (sweeping hands) or bhujangasana (sweeping hands)

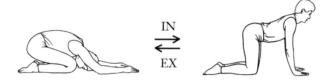

Chakravakasana

2. Shalamba Sarvangasana (Shoulderstand)

shalamba - supported   *sarvanga* - all parts

The Classical Posture

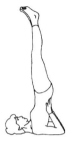

Head and shoulders are on the floor, facing upward.
The trunk and leg form a vertical, straight line.
The legs are straight, and the feet are together.
The upper arms and elbows are on the floor, parallel
to each other, with the hands supporting the trunk
from the back.

The Modified Version

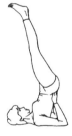

The position of the arms may be modified.
The legs can be slightly bent, and one can
begin from a bent knee position.

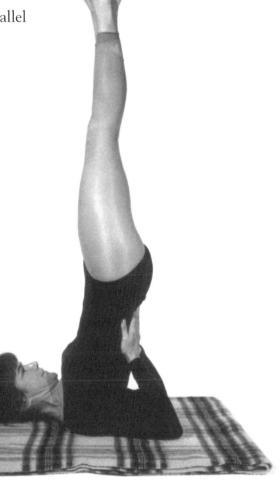

Vinyasa Krama

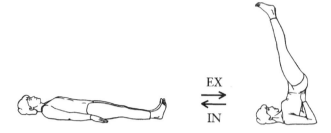

Begin lying on the floor, your arms by your sides and your legs together. Lift your head slightly, to check that your body is correctly aligned, then return your head to the floor.

On the exhale, lift your legs toward your head allowing your torso to lift off the ground at the same time. Bring your hands to your lower back above your buttocks to support the torso.

As you return to the ground, slightly bend your knees and gently lower your torso to the floor, without lifting your head from the floor.

Notes

Do not insist on keeping your elbows parallel, as this may produce tension in your neck.

Balancing Posture

The balancing postures are the same as *viparita karani*.

3. Shalamba Shirshasana (Headstand)

shalamba - supported   *shirsha* - head

The Classical Posture

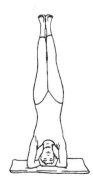 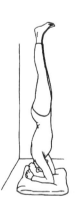

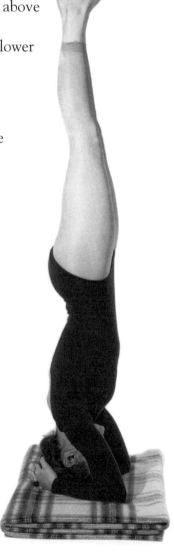

The body is held straight, with the head aligned normally with the spine.

The elbows and forearms are on the floor, with the fingers interlocked behind the head.

The upper arms are parallel.

The legs are straight, the feet together.

The Modified Version

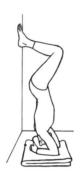

The knees may be bent to release pressure on the back and to allow the abdomen to stay relaxed.

The legs may separate, thereby insuring the stability that allows for comfortable and relaxed breathing.

The feet and toes may also relax to decrease tension that can inhibit smooth breathing.

The knees may be bent while moving into and out of the posture, to reduce stress on the back and neck.

The elbows may also be spread further apart, if necessary, to insure easy balance. The distance between them will be contingent upon the muscular development of the shoulders and upper back.

Note: Remember *never* to make adjustments while *in* the headstand. Instead, come down and repeat the posture, preferably with the guidance of a teacher.

Vinyasa Krama

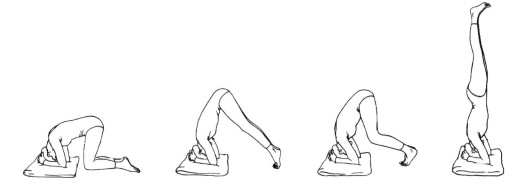

Beginning on hands and knees, interlock your fingers, leaving the thumbs up to support your head. Look backwards between your arms to check that your feet are aligned evenly between the elbows.

On the inhale, lift your hips. Straighten your legs, keep the feet touching the floor. On the exhale, bend your knees and bring your feet near your torso. On the inhale, bring your legs upward to a vertical position.

To come down, on the exhale bend your knees and lower your body back to the starting position.

Note: It is particularly important that the sequencing leading up to, and out of, shirshasana be carefully planned and carried out. Please refer to the chapter on sequencing for examples of this process.

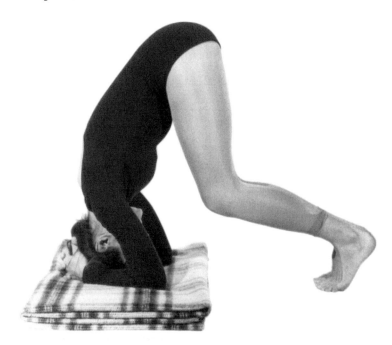

Learning Stages

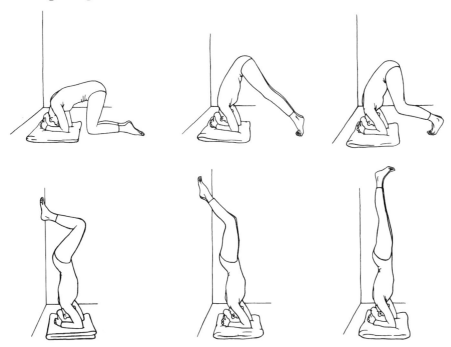

Initially, use the wall for support so that a single direction is supported. (A corner supports two directions and is confusing.)

Beginning on your hands and knees, interlock your fingers, leaving the thumbs up to support your head. Place your head in your hands, about six inches from the wall.

Note: If you are right up against the wall, all your weight will rest against the wall. If your alignment is not right, the stress will be transferred to your neck, and may lead to numbness in your fingers.

Line up your elbows and feet, as shown in the drawing above. On the inhale, straighten your knees so that you lift your hips. On the exhale, bend your knees and walk your feet inward toward your head.

Press your knees and kick up to the wall, leaving your knees bent. Feel the wall, hold for one normal breath, steady yourself, and then walk the feet up the wall. Press your elbows down evenly. Allow your feet to separate slightly.

To come down, on the exhale bend your knees and lower your body back to the starting position.

Notes

The ideal head position will differ according to the shape of the head. If the head position is not correct, it is likely that the weight will be unevenly distributed and the tendency will be to press with the elbows to compensate for this imbalance. You should support the head with all the fingers, including the little fingers pressed slightly under the head and the thumbs directed upward along the sides of the head.

The base of the headstand is comprised of the head and elbows. Ideally, the weight supported by the head and each elbow should be the same, and the three should form an equilateral triangle. If the weight is too much toward the back of the body, the stress is transferred up through the shoulders to the neck. Move your body to shift the weight to your elbows rather than allowing it to stay on your neck, which is much more fragile. Do not, however, place all of your weight on your elbows.

It is also not advisable to do headstand with props that allow the neck to hang freely; the weight of the head and the psychological inhibition will cause one's neck muscles to contract.

Ideally, the body will be perfectly vertical and symmetrical in the headstand. It is therefore important to note where asymmetry exists while one is inverted. This will require the help of another person, as it is not possible to see yourself from all the necessary angles — even with a mirror. Remember, again, that you should *never* adjust the posture while in it. You must instead come down and reposition yourself, making the adjustments when moving back into the position.

Balancing Postures

The shoulderstand is often considered the traditional balancing pose for headstand because it reverses the backbending and neck curvature. However, viparita karani is safer and can be used instead.

It is advisable to rest your neck before attempting the balancing posture. Also, after coming out of headstand, lie on your back and rest to relax your neck and lower back before doing other balancing postures.

Vinyasa Krama for Balancing

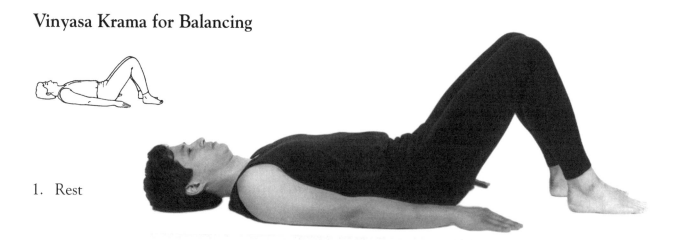

1. Rest

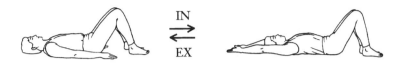

2. Arm raises

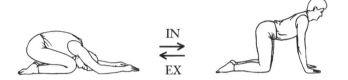

3. Chakravakasana

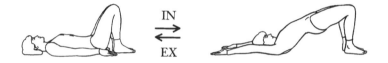

4. Dvipada pitham with arms

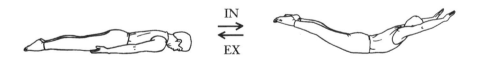

5. Shalabhasana

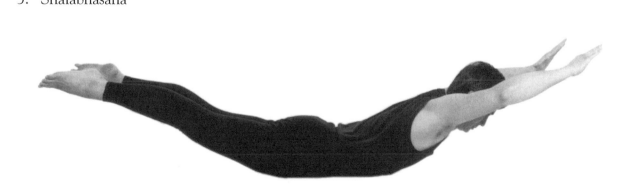

The headstand must be planned as part of a vinyasa krama that deals with preparation and balancing for it. In addition, you must remain sensitive to fatigue, as well as to emotional or structural difficulties that occur as the practice progresses.

In such cases, it may be necessary to add appropriate rests or transitional postures, to eliminate some postures, or even to alter the final goal. In this way each posture is meaningful in the practice, and the overall intention is fulfilled.

5

VINYASA KRAMA — SEQUENCING AND ADAPTATION

The Importance of Vinyasa Krama

The order in which the poses are done in an asana practice is not an arbitrary matter. You may have all the right ingredients for a powerful practice, but if they are poorly ordered you not only won't achieve your goal, you will also stand a chance of hurting yourself.

It is as if the asanas were the letters of the alphabet. When strung together without purpose they form nonsense, but when properly ordered they create words, sentences, and wondrous literature. Each asana can have a different effect depending on the steps leading up to it and those that follow. Any posture can be beneficial or harmful depending on these factors.

Earlier we discussed vinyasa krama — the intelligent ordering of postures to achieve a goal. Vinyasa krama is also known as "sequencing." It is the practical means for attaining steadiness (sthira) and comfort (sukha). To create an effective sequence you will need to:

- Start out with a clear purpose or goal.
- Make the adaptations necessary to accomplishing that purpose, according to your individual capacity and limits.
- Adjust the sequence so that it fits into the time you have available.
- Use the breath and inner attention as feedback to determine if you are doing the best sequence to accomplish your goal.

In addition, you must consider:

1. The characteristics of your goal. If your goal is to do a headstand, for instance, you need to see what parts of the body will be involved, so that you can properly prepare them. In headstand, the back and neck must bear weight and the body will be inverted, so your breathing will be affected. This means that you must observe these areas to see if they can support the posture adequately, and also gently prepare them for doing the posture.

Preparatory postures will often fulfill both purposes. For example, a standing forward bend will demonstrate the strength and flexibility of the back, as well as warm it up for doing headstand. A twist will show whether the neck can be supportive and weight-bearing, and will also warm the area through the movement.

2. What activities precede your practice. For example, it is not advisable to exercise heavily before asana practice. If you run or do aerobics before you practice, you may find that a strong forward bend (such as a seated forward bend) may cause cramps and that your legs will shake during the standing postures. Therefore, the purpose of your practice will not be effectively met.

3. What activities will follow your practice. What you do after your practice will determine the state in which you will want to end your sequence. For example, if you plan to sleep immediately afterward, doing many active postures will counteract this purpose. Relaxing breathing techniques will be more effective.

There are four major elements of sequencing: Preparation, Balancing, Rest, and Ending. We will discuss them in turn.

1. Preparation

Each pose you do will require adequate preparation. This means that you will need a progression of postures and movements to warm up your muscles and loosen your joints. The following are general guidelines:

- Begin with the easy and progress to the more difficult postures.

Easy   Difficult

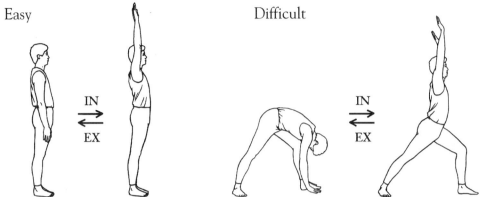

IN
EX

IN
EX

- Begin with the known and progress to the unknown — that is, start
  out with movements your body already knows how to do, and go
  from there into movements that are unfamiliar or foreign to it.

Known   Unknown

Used to   Not used to

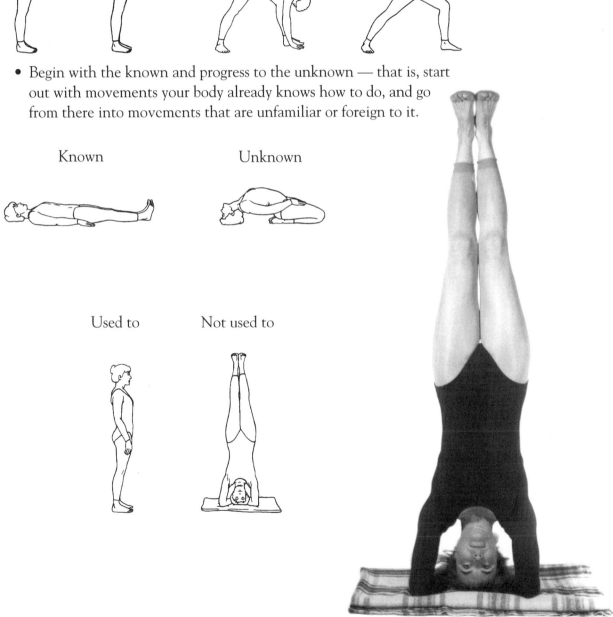

- Begin by moving in and out of postures, and progress to staying in them.

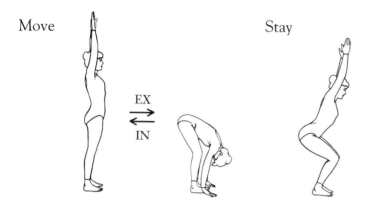

These guidelines apply to all aspects of a practice — from preparing for one pose, to planning an entire sequence.

How to Begin Your Practice

We will now go on to look more closely at the best way to begin any particular sequence. It is best to begin from a position that is easy, familiar, and consistent with your present condition. This includes the physical, mental, and situational components.

- For an early morning practice after a sound sleep, a standing posture is a good beginning.

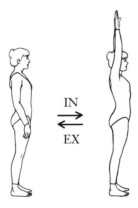

- An evening practice intended for relaxation may begin in a seated or lying position.

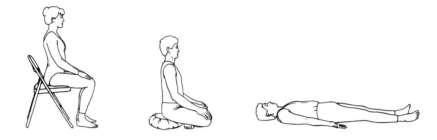

- If your body is already warmed up, you may begin with simple forward bending movements.

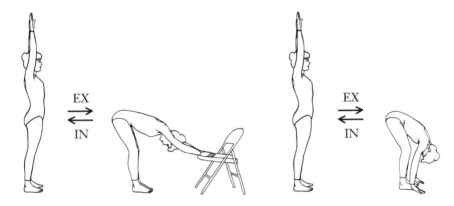

- Simple arm movement is an ideal beginning for a practice. This movement warms up the back and demonstrates the condition of the neck and shoulders, which are common areas of tension and pain. Done correctly, this movement involves the breath and gently moves the entire spine. It also includes upward and downward motion. See the examples on page 130.

  In addition, when done with deep conscious breathing, this simple arm movement provides the opportunity for self-observation and awareness that must become a continual part of every asana practice. You need to be aware of stiffness in your body, tension in any area, and the state of your breath throughout your practice, so that you can make any necessary modifications.

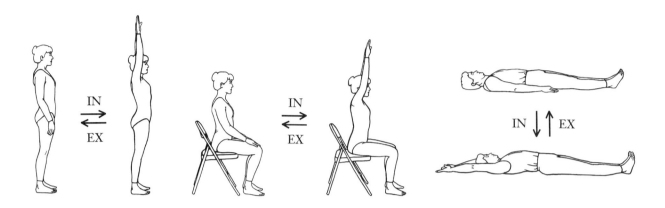

- The first part of your practice should consist of forward bending movements because the body is used to performing them. Most daily activities such as sitting, driving, working at a desk, lifting, and so on, involve forward bending. Forward bends allow the body to transition easily into asanas that take more effort, change, or learning.

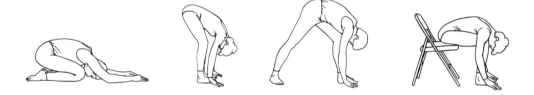

- You may also begin with a simple vinyasa that brings about movement in the spine.

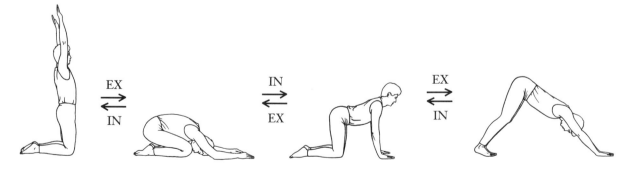

It is unwise to begin your practice with:

Deep arches

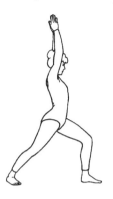 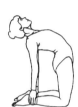

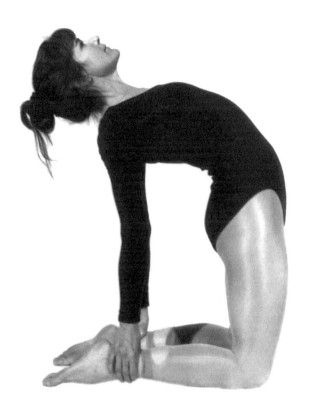

Twists

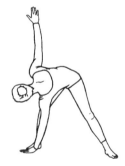 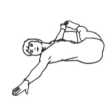

Headstand or shoulderstand

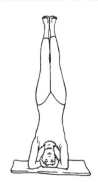 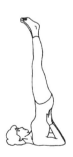

Static postures   Lateral bends   Difficult postures

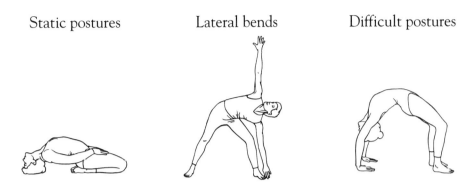

The body must be warmed up and gradually led into the more difficult postures.

It is also important to learn the preparatory postures first so that the body will be properly conditioned for the final pose. For example, before you can do a difficult posture like the wheel, you should prepare and strengthen your back.

It is therefore necessary to be able to perform shalabhasana (locust), and to be able to stay in it for several breaths. Although it is a less difficult posture, it uses and thus strengthens the same parts of the body as the wheel.

If locust is not comfortable for you, you may try cobra, which is a preparation for locust. Indeed, both of these poses must be mastered before doing the final posture.

Cobra   Locust   Wheel

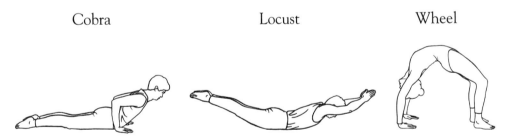

To sum up, in preparation for a particular asana you should use a sequence of similar, but less difficult, postures. There are many such preparatory stages for any given asana. Also, what is difficult for one student will be easy for another. Therefore, it is important that teachers recognize the abilities of their students and teach each posture over the appropriate period of time and in the correct order.

Preparing the Breath

To prepare for a posture you must also prepare for the breathing you will use in it. For example:

Uttanasana stretches the back and prepares the body for breathing in an inverted position. To prepare for static inversions such as headstand or viparita karani, one should be able to stay in uttanasana for several breaths and breathe comfortably.

Dvipada pitham prepares the neck and the breath, and is preparation for inversion. If the breathing is difficult in this posture, do not attempt inversion.

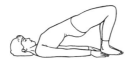

Moving in the Posture as Preparation for Staying in It

Generally, staying in a posture is more difficult than moving in and out of it, although there are exceptions such as the headstand. Therefore, the preparation should reflect that difficulty and adequately prepare you for this difference.

Preparing to Stay in Chair Pose

If, for example, your goal is to stay in chair pose (ardha utkatasana) for six breaths, you must first master the following steps:

- You must be able to repeat the posture without problems.

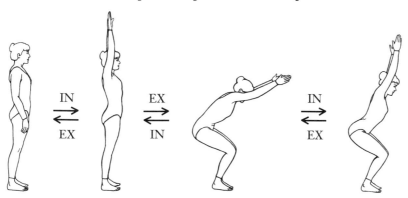

- Strong knees are essential to this posture, so you must be able to do and repeat the squatting posture.

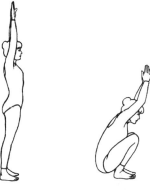

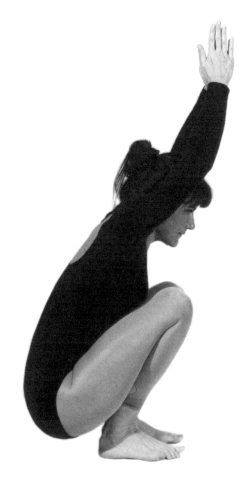

- You must be able to stay in a similar posture, such as ardha uttanasana.

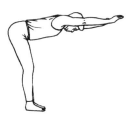

Preparing for Headstand

Dvipada pitham

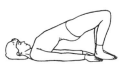

Uttanasana

Standing twist

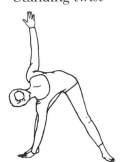

Leg raises

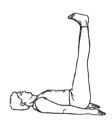

Shalabhasana

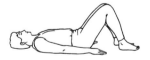

- Before attempting headstand or shoulderstand, check the condition of the back and neck using a twisting posture.

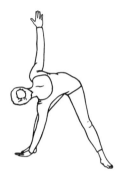

- Do not attempt headstand immediately after a posture such as leg raises that stresses the abdomen.

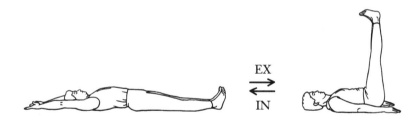

- Rest and relax the legs before doing headstand.

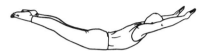

2. Balancing Postures

After a difficult pose your body will naturally feel inclined to move or stretch in a way that compensates for the effort made. This is simply the body's way of balancing itself. For example, after practicing shalabhasana — whether holding it or repeating it — most people will enjoy the action of bringing the knees in toward the chest.

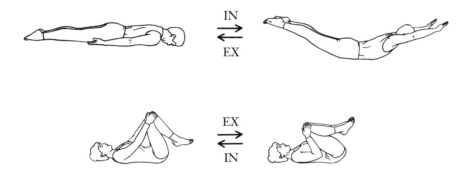

This action removes the resistance (tightness in the back, neck, or shoulders) caused by the previous position. It balances the effect of the previous asana. The Sanskrit word used for such a balancing posture is *pratikriyasana*, which means "opposite action or movement." It does not necessarily mean opposite posture.

The process of following an asana with a completely reversed configuration can be harmful. This is therefore not the correct way to balance your practice. For example, the opposite posture of headstand is standing upright, which is not suitable after inversion. The opposite posture for wheel is a seated forward bend (paschimatanasana) which, for many, can be a strenuous posture in its own right, and does not relieve the areas of tension created in the first one. While fish is traditionally used to balance shoulderstand, it may be harmful, for it stresses the neck just after it has been severely stretched.

Activity and relaxation work together to maintain one's overall balance and integration. Relaxation will balance one activity and prepare for the next. Similarly, a balancing posture should release tension and restore balance in the area used in one posture, even as it leads gently toward the next one. In correct sequencing each asana serves both these purposes, thus creating a smooth and balanced course that becomes an integrating experience for the student.

The examples on page 138 illustrate ways in which an asana can both balance one posture and prepare for another.

Pose	Preparation	Balance
1) Arm Raises IN ⇄ EX	Preparation for uttanasana (2).	Raising and lowering arms are balancing movements to each other. Raising arms is a mild arch. Lowering them is a release of the arch.
2) Uttanasana IN ⇄ EX	Prepares the body for viparita karani (4) by stretching the neck and back. Prepares breathing for inversion.	This is a forward movement that can balance both back-bends and twists.
3) Dvipada pitham IN ⇄ EX	Prepares the body for viparita karani (4) by both inversion and stretching the neck. If you cannot stay and breathe in this, do not attempt viparita karani.	Balances uttanasana (2).
4) Viparita karani	Preparation for plough pose (halasana) — not shown here. Increases lightness in the legs. In this sequence it is the main pose.	Can be a balance for headstand (not shown here).
5) Bhujangasana IN ⇄ EX	Preparation for locust (shalabhasana) — not shown here.	Balances Viparita karani (4).
6) Vajrasana EX ⇄ IN	A preparatory pose for uttanasana.	This balances bhujangasana.
7) Shavasana	This posture (shavasana) can be a prep or a principle posture for considerations like hypertension.	This balances vajrasana.

General Principles for Balancing Your Practice

- Balancing postures should be mild in comparison to the preceding posture.
- Balancing postures should involve movement. Usually this means that you will be repeating the balancing posture, moving in and out of it.
- Rest is a balancing posture. If you are in doubt about the correct balancing posture for the preceding posture, simply rest. Indeed, it is advisable to intersperse rest between other postures in order to balance your practice. This will naturally prolong the length of the session, so you must be sure to allow enough time for a proper ending.

  Rest periods are also good times for self-observation. You may examine the effect of the previous posture while you rest, and make any necessary modifications to your program. This kind of feedback is an integral part of any meaningful asana practice.
- Sometimes it may be necessary to use two postures for balancing. The first one may be a resting position. For example:

After headstand:

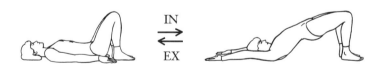

Rest

1.

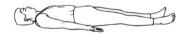

2.

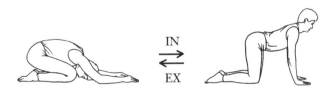

After shalabhasana:

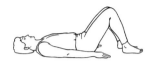

Rest

1.

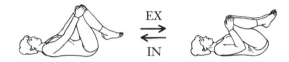

EX

IN

2.

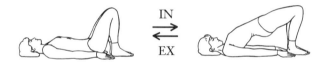

IN

EX

- Use a symmetrical forward bend to prepare for, and to balance, a twist.

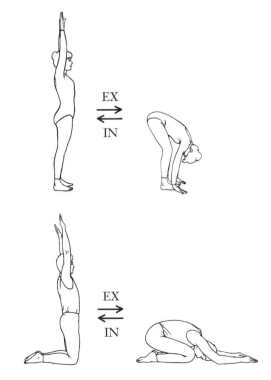

- Learn the balancing posture *before* learning the posture it is
  to balance.

Learn this	Before

Note: There are also other balancing postures that may be used in these cases.

- Use a balancing posture between two difficult postures. This will enable you to perform the second posture with renewed strength and vitality, preventing possible injury from fatigue.

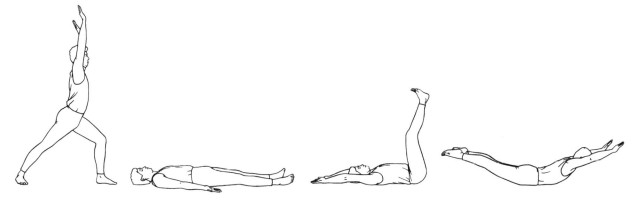

3. Rest

Rest is an extremely important component of asana practice. It is perhaps the most crucial aspect of the practice in terms of personal reintegration. During rest you can observe yourself and become directly aware of the link between body, breath, and mind. When the body, breath, or attention tires, the link between them changes. During rest a centering and reunification of these elements takes place. The disharmony is eliminated and all parts of the person may then move in an integrated fashion. Rest, therefore, is not a passive break in your practice, but an active and important part of the process of reintegration.

There are several other functions that rest provides during a practice. Most obviously, when you rest, you get your energy back. This lets you perform the next asana with vitality and full attention. Rest can also serve as a balancing posture in a routine where the postures get more difficult as the practice moves along. In this instance, rest will assure that a student is as capable and balanced in the final position as in the first.

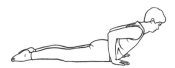 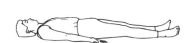 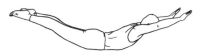

In a successful asana practice you should be able to breathe easily. Rest
serves an important role in making this happen. When either your mind or
body becomes tired your breath will indicate the fatigue. Rest will restore
normal breathing so that your practice may continue with body, breath, and
mind functioning as one.

There is no standard format about exactly when or how long to rest. It
depends on the individual. Many people feel that rest is appropriate when
working muscles become sore or fatigued and the body no longer performs as
it did at the beginning of practice. In fact, however, this is too late, for it
means that the body has been working without the full support of correct
breath and an attentive mind.

The best indicator of when to rest is the breath. When the breath is no
longer smooth and long, it is time to rest. This is particularly easy to detect
when you practice ujjayi, or "throat" breathing, while doing asanas. This
method of breathing (described in Chapter 2) constricts the throat in a way
that produces an actual sound. When your mind is focused, any change or
break in the smooth, controlled sound of the breath is obvious. This serves
as a sign that you need to rest in order to reintegrate body, breath, and mind.

As mentioned above, the amount of rest necessary varies according to
each student, activity, or situation. The two main guidelines are breath and
energy. Rest until your breath returns to normal and your energy is fully
replenished.

The following are some of the resting postures that you can bring into
your practice:

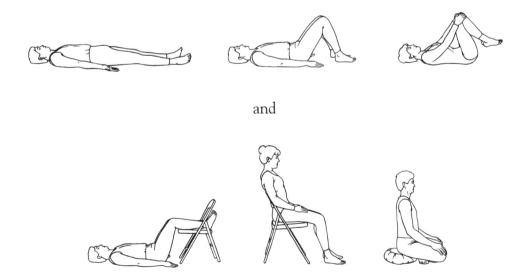

and

4. Ending Your Practice

The overall effect of a practice is determined by the *entire* sequence. Therefore, the ending of a session deserves careful attention, because it can significantly affect the transition into your next activity, and heighten or lessen the intended effect of the practice as a whole. The aim is to end in a state that helps sustain the integration of body, mind, and breath throughout your succeeding activities and in your general, daily life.

The end of the asana practice bears some similarities to its beginning. Thus, the final posture should be mild and simple.

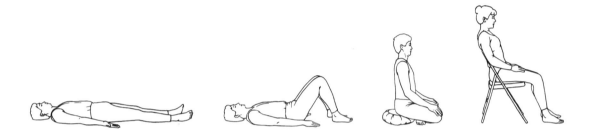

This is why it is not a good idea to end a session with a headstand, backbend, intense forward bend, twist, or lateral bend, such as:

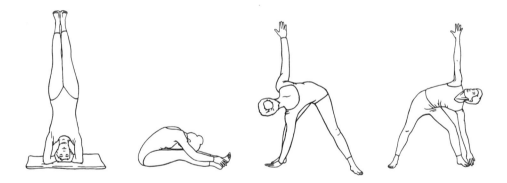

Sequencing for Individual Needs

Correct sequencing is both an art and a science. It is a complex matter involving a knowledge of the principles, clear and continuous self-assessment, prior organization, and considerable creativity. For every goal there are many paths. For every person there are many possible practices. For every practice there are an enormous number of variables that have an impact on its effect. However, consideration of all these factors will result in a truly integrative practice.

Following are illustrations of various courses for a single purpose: to increase the feeling of lightness in one's legs. However, the courses vary according to many factors. We use this example to demonstrate two points:

1. How different a course needs to be for different people — even when they all share the same purpose.
2. How different a course needs to be for the same person at different times of day.

Case 1

Person: Young (30 years old), athletic and active, practices yoga regularly.
Purpose: Lightness in the legs
Time of Day: Morning
Condition: Fresh
Preceding activity: Sleep
Time available: Forty minutes
Succeeding activity: Work

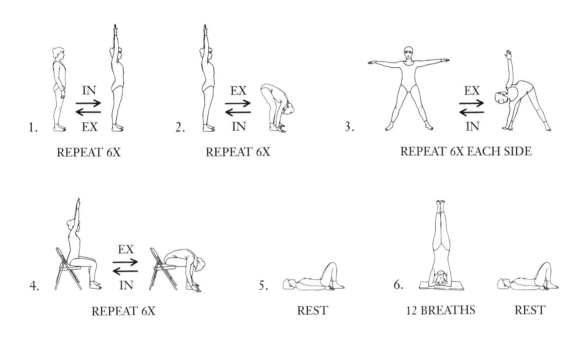

1. REPEAT 6X 2. REPEAT 6X 3. REPEAT 6X EACH SIDE

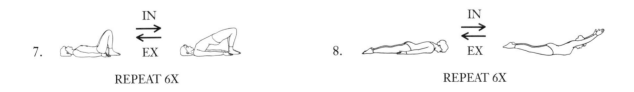

4. REPEAT 6X 5. REST 6. 12 BREATHS REST

7. REPEAT 6X 8. REPEAT 6X

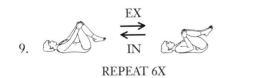 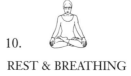

9. REPEAT 6X 10. REST & BREATHING

Case 2

Person: Same
Purpose: Same
Time of day: Evening
Condition: Tired
Time available: Fifteen minutes
Succeeding activities: Eating and sleeping

1. 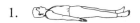 STAY
12 BREATHS

2. 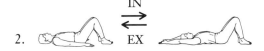 REPEAT 6X

3. 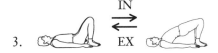 REPEAT 6X

4. 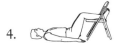 STAY
12 BREATHS   LONG EXHALE

5. 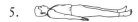 REST 2 MIN.

Case 3

Person: Older, (65 years), stiff back and legs, cannot do headstand or shoulderstand.
Purpose: Lightness in the legs
Time of day: Evening
Condition: Tired
Time available: Fifteen minutes
Succeeding activities: Eating and sleeping

1. 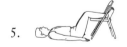   12 BREATHS

2. 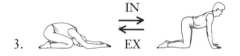   REPEAT 6X EACH SIDE

3. 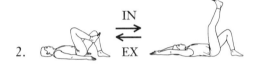   REPEAT 6X

4. 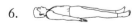   REST 2 MIN.

5. 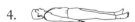   12 BREATHS

6. 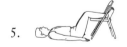   REST 2 MIN.

7. 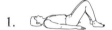   12 BREATHS

The goal of your practice may be to learn a new asana. The following four sequences show examples of classes that will thoroughly prepare you to perform locust pose (shalabhasana) over a period of time.

Sequence One

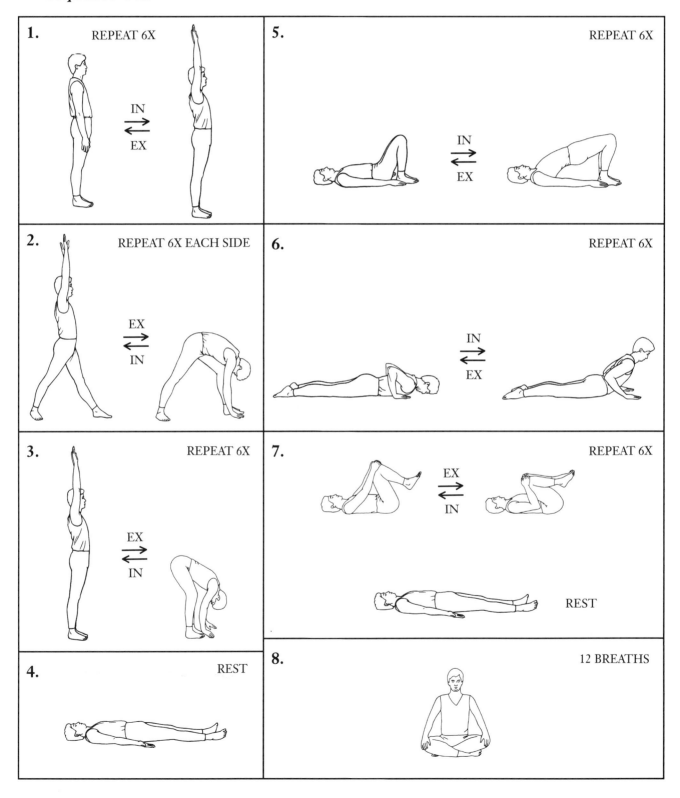

Sequence Two

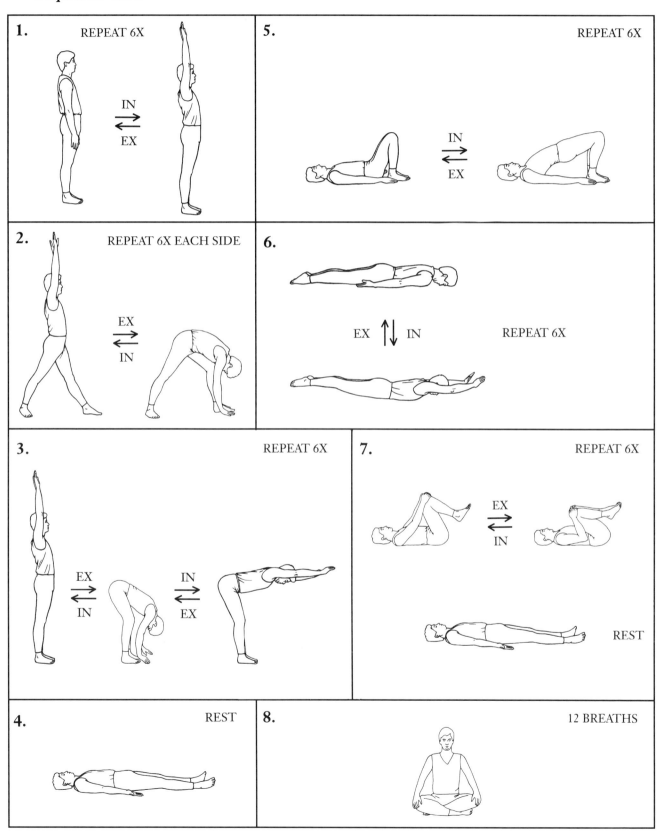

Sequence Three

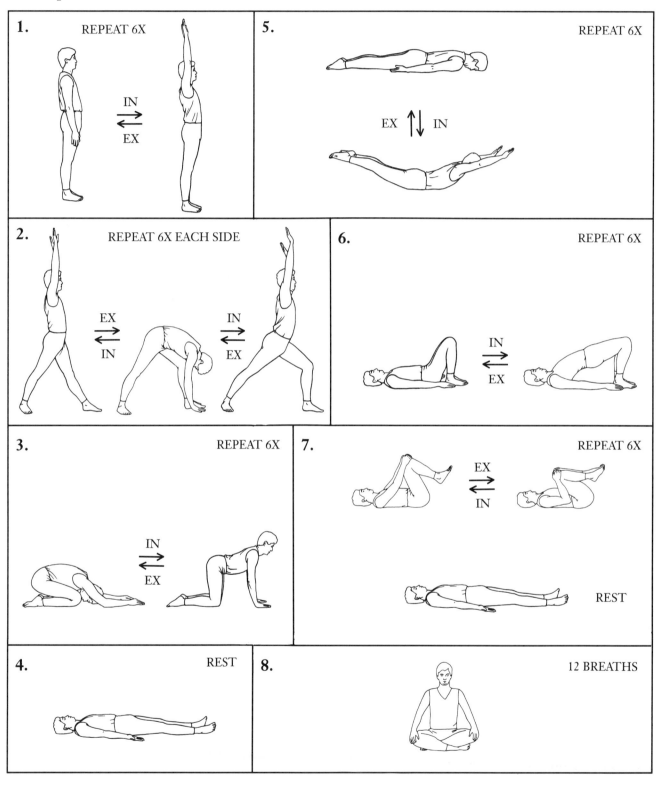

Sequence Four

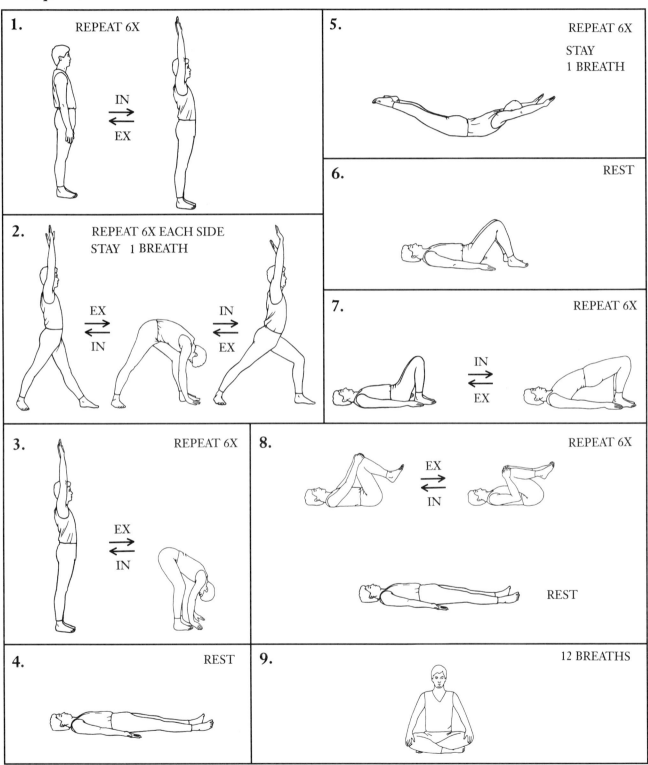

Considerations in Sequence Planning

Age

You can practice yoga at any age, as long as your practice is done correctly. You simply need to evaluate the feasibility of your goals according to your age. Your practice must also reflect your physical and mental capabilities and limitations.

Although the elderly and the young should not be doing the same practice, there is no reason why their respective practices can't be equally productive and rewarding. In general, the proportion of a practice devoted to reflection will increase with age. Children will spend little, if any, time in quiet meditation or breathing techniques, while the elderly will perhaps devote the majority of their practice to these aspects. For their purposes, simple arm movements and gentle breathing done in a standing, sitting, or lying position can be very effective.

For children, asana should be growth-oriented. An asana practice for children should include dynamic postures which demand agility and are somewhat challenging. Children like to practice in groups, where healthy competition develops an excitement and interest that will aid the momentum of learning. Often, the postures are strung together in a sequence to keep the students' attention. At this age the attention span is relatively short, and long periods of instruction or talking are boring. Concentration is then lost. It is therefore best to keep children physically active, directing their seemingly boundless energy into areas that are both useful and enjoyable for them, helping them grow.

Sound or chanting can also help to consciously coordinate breath and movement in the asanas. Often coordinated with movement, sound facilitates the linkage necessary for reintegration without undue mental effort and possible frustration. Included below are some examples of appropriate sequences for children.

Children's Vinyasa for Navasana

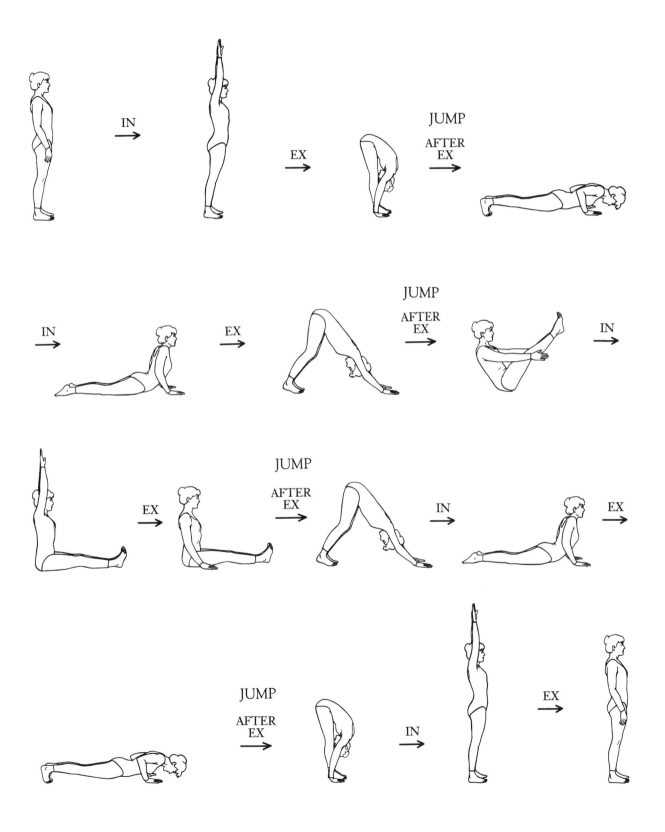

Children's Vinyasa for Paschimatanasana
(Seated Forward Bend)

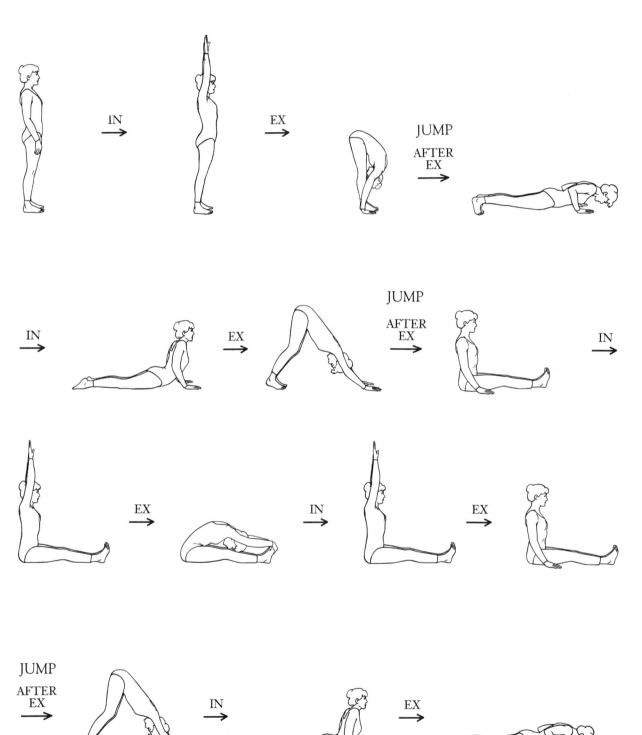

Children's Vinyasas, continued

JUMP

AFTER
EX
$\longrightarrow$

IN
$\longrightarrow$

EX
$\longrightarrow$

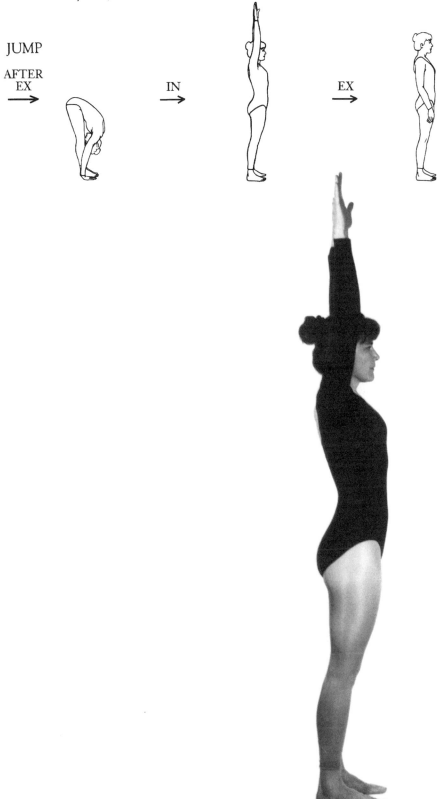

Gender: Women's Considerations

The appropriate practice during pregnancy, menstruation, and menopause must be determined on an individual basis. In pregnancy, for example, it is advisable that a woman consult with her physician and coordinate her practice with a yoga teacher. Some factors that should be considered are whether or not she regularly practiced yoga before her pregnancy, whether or not she has suffered any miscarriages, and whether or not she has any specific ailments or structural difficulties such as asthma, back problems, and so on.

In general, if a woman *does* practice during pregnancy, it is advisable to avoid pressure on the abdomen.

Simple postures that include comfortable breathing can be beneficial. Normally, practice can begin in the fourth month of pregnancy and continue until delivery, as long as the practice is modified appropriately as time progresses.

Asana can most certainly be useful during both menstruation and menopause so long as one's preferences, limitations, and the continual feedback from self-observation is carefully taken into account. Generally, mild exercise and breathing are more useful than difficult and complex postures.

Level of Experience

You may begin yoga without any related experience or knowledge. It is not necessary to be able to stand on your head, sit in a lotus position, or hold your breath for prolonged periods of time.

With skillful instruction, observation, and an awareness of the intended goal, an appropriate practice can be designed for anyone, regardless of their age, ability, or level of experience.

Weight

Prosperity and a sedentary life style have many side effects, overweight being a common one. For people with this condition, yoga can be extremely beneficial in terms of the exercise itself and the resulting state of mind, both of which are components in helping to bring about weight loss.

For overweight students, some adaptations to postures are necessary. For instance, a large belly can be a hindrance in postures such as deep forward bends. It is important that the teacher give adaptations and eliminate the more difficult postures, so that the student will have a positive experience. Otherwise, a practice that is awkward or too difficult may do damage to an already low self-esteem.

Fitness

Yoga is an excellent means for maintaining a high level of physical conditioning. Depending on the design of a practice, it can help to develop muscular strength and endurance, flexibility, and cardiovascular capacity. The level of intensity can be changed according to a student's condition and aspirations.

Yoga for Athletes

Yoga is helpful to athletes in several ways. First, it is helpful before an athletic event in reducing the mental tension that could adversely affect performance. It is also effective after the event for relaxation purposes.

In addition, a corrective asana program can be therapeutic for treating injuries and overuse syndromes that result from certain activities. It is, of course, also quite useful in balancing the muscular system and conditioning the body, mind, and breath to perform optimally in any situation, whether it be athletic or not. The point to note is that when asana is combined with other forms of exercise, it is advisable to allow a sufficient gap of time between them, so that each can performed with full attention, energy, and muscular capability.

Diet: Vegetarianism and Fasting

While food has a definite effect on one's health and ability to function, vegetarianism is not a prerequisite for the practice of yoga. In fact, vegetarian food that includes many deep-fried dishes could be less healthy than a non-vegetarian diet. A normal, healthy diet is recommended.

The *Yoga Sutras* advise moderation in all things. The Sanskrit word for fasting is *upa vasa*. Upa means "near," and vas means "to dwell." The purpose of fasting is for the mind to stay, or dwell, near God. A fast should increase one's alertness and help him or her to focus inside. Asana practice should be modified during a fast to reflect the difference in one's energy level and physical strength. The practice may be continued with a single day's fast, but the student should carefully consider whether continuing over a number of days is really appropriate.

For some people and in certain situations, fasting may cause mental disturbances. In such instances, it is not advised. In cases where the mind dwells on food rather than on God, one will not achieve positive results.

Lifestyle and Health

It is not necessary to give up smoking and drinking in order to practice yoga, because trying to suppress or give up habits as a prerequisite to practice may only result in increased mental tension. However, one of the results of a correct practice is that one is changed on many levels. Practice tends to weaken unhealthy habits and enhance healthy ones. Frequently, this paves the way for a change in habits such as smoking, drinking, or drug use.

All of these factors should be taken into account in planning one's practice. While it may seem as though this makes the planning of a practice quite complicated, in fact it does not. Rather, you learn to put together a practice that is a direct response both to your current situation and to the goals you have determined. This is the true way to create a practice that is ultimately beneficial.

6

PRANAYAMA — THE ROLE OF BREATH IN PERSONAL REINTEGRATION

This chapter deals exclusively with the breath, or pranayama. Pranayama is a central component in the theory and practice of yoga. Of the eight limbs of yoga listed by Patanjali in the *Yoga Sutras*, it is one of the three that provide actual techniques for practice. For this reason, pranayama, along with asana, is an accessible method with which to start a yoga practice and thereby begin a path toward personal reintegration. It has therefore been widely discussed in both ancient and modern yoga literature.

The meaning of the word pranayama can be confusing. It is often mistakenly thought to be composed of *prana* and *yama* (control), and is thus understood to mean "control of the breath." However, pranayama is to be understood as *prana* and *ayama* (to lengthen, stretch, extend.) Prana is a concept that means "life force." The prefix *pra* means "very well" and *an* means "to go" or "to travel." Prana, then, is that which travels well through all parts of the body, inside us. It is the total energy that makes up a human being, entering at birth and leaving at death. It is responsible for the function of life: The improper flow of prana is illness and the absence of prana is death.

Prana exists in all living things. We cannot acquire more prana from the outside — by breathing it into our bodies, for instance. Rather, it resides within us and, when allowed to flow correctly, results in ideal functioning. The concept of prana is also used in Ayurveda, an ancient system of health maintenance.

Prana is responsible for all functions of life: the physiological systems such as the cardiovascular, digestive, endocrine systems, and so on, as well as the mind and the senses. It is linked to consciousness. When your mind focuses on your hand, for instance, prana is the force behind that focus. Ideally, it should be centered and flowing in a single, desired direction. When one's life force is scattered by food, thoughts, activities, and so on, the body and mind are negatively affected. Breath is not prana, although the two are commonly thought to be the same. Nor is prana air. If it were, then pumping air into a dead body would revive it. Rather, breath is the *expression* of prana, the expression of life and the force behind it. While prana cannot be seen, touched, or directly manipulated, the breath is a sort of lever, or method, for working on it indirectly. So, when the breath is affected, prana is also affected, because the two are directly related.

As we have seen in earlier chapters, the goal of yoga is to direct the activities of the mind so that it can see more clearly. This requires that you must first remove impurities. This purification is accomplished through pranayama. In fact, pranayama is regarded as the greatest of all cleansing methods, and is included in all Hindu rituals for this reason. When practiced correctly, its positive results can be extremely significant, deeply affecting the individual on many levels. Moreover, given the close association of body, breath, and mind, breath can and should be used as an effective means of working with the body. If yoga is a tool of reflection, pranayama may be seen as a means of sharpening this tool.

There are many fallacious assumptions associated with the theory of pranayama. Pranayama is not the awakening of the coiled serpent. Nor is its purpose to produce levitation, to come out alive after being buried for days, to hold one's breath as long as possible, or to practice difficult and obscure breathing ratios. Rather, pranayama is the conscious regulation of the breath. When you practice it, you deliberately change your normal pattern of breathing which, in turn, changes your state of mind. This reduces mental disturbance, and minimizes the impurities in your system. As a result, you become clearer and your understanding is enhanced. The ultimate aim of pranayama, then, is to focus the mind.

The Removal of Impurities

The impurities that exist in our systems are subtle, existing inside everyone, but invisible to those who possess them. Although they may be considered primarily mental in nature, the *Yoga Sutras* does not differentiate between physical and mental impurities. In this text, the only word used to describe them is *asuddhi*, meaning "that which is not clean, which should not be in the system, or which is in a place where it does not belong."

Pranayama is considered to be the highest of the *tapas*, which literally means "to cook." Just as the proper cooking of food enables the body to take it in, assimilating from it what it needs and eliminating what it doesn't need, pranayama both enables the mind to focus on a chosen object (PYS II:53) and to remove the impurities that cloud clear perception (PYS II:52). It thus cleanses the mind to prepare it for focusing on a desired object.

According to yoga texts, "fire" (agni) exists inside our bodies near the navel. The impurities settle below that, in the abdominal area called *apana*. This fire burns impurities, and our breath affects the quality of the flame. Furthermore, breath regulates the flow of impurities toward the fire for burning, and away from it in order to leave the body. Various breathing patterns, which will be discussed later in the chapter, can be used for this process.

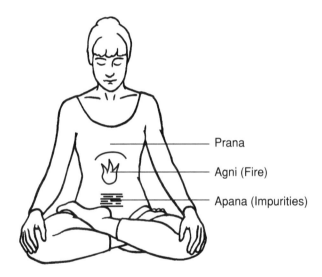

Prana

Agni (Fire)

Apana (Impurities)

Pranayama leaves the mind in a state where meditation, or absorption, is possible. With a clear mind, you can fix your attention steadily on a subject of your choice. Without the proper preparation of pranayama, meditation may involve only the imagination. This may be enjoyable, but it is not the intended goal. The ultimate goal for this breathing practice is to change your state of mind, allowing it to focus on a subject that will lead you closer to personal reintegration.

The correct practice of pranayama also brings about another powerful effect. Earlier we stated that all things possess all three gunas: the qualities of lightness or clarity (satva), dullness or heaviness (tamas), and excitement or activity (rajas). All three are necessary, but at any specific time you want the appropriate balance between them, in order to facilitate whatever you are doing at the moment.

For example, it is not ideal to be predominantly rajasic at bedtime or tamasic when it is time to start working. When one guna is increased, the others decrease. The extent to which any of these is present is affected by one's diet, thoughts, and activities. Through various types of practice, we can replace one dominant guna with another, such that we can respond appropriately to the present moment. Moreover, pranayama increases satva, so that the mind is clear and in a state of focus.

Conscious Breathing

The *Yoga Sutras* (II:49) defines pranayama as the conscious changing of one's breathing pattern. You must do this in a comfortable posture so that all your attention can be focused on your breathing pattern without distraction.

Changes that occur in your breathing during running or singing, for example, are not pranayama, because they are simply a result of these activities.

In conscious breathing we are aware of the breathing process and are therefore able to purposely affect it. In sleep we are unconscious of everything. Even when awake or conscious during the day, we are generally unconscious of our breathing pattern. In becoming aware of the nature of our breathing, we become able to regulate or change it over a period of time, usually several cycles of the breath.

Why the emphasis on conscious or deliberate breathing? Although we spend our entire lives breathing, we are generally not conscious of doing so. By consciously regulating our breath, we also consciously link the breath and the mind, thereby bringing about a change in our minds. This change in pattern reduces disturbances of the mind so that it can focus more easily. As we lessen the disturbances of our minds, we reduce our misperceptions and heighten our understanding. We can then achieve the ultimate aim of yoga.

Once you are conscious of your breath, this regulation can either be a matter of passively observing it, or actively modulating it. In passive observation, you link the mind to the breath, but do not regulate it. You simply remain aware of the quality of the breath — its inhale, exhale, and the pauses between the two. You do not attempt to change any of these characteristics; you merely focus on the present nature of your breath.

You can experiment with this yourself. Without making any actual change in your breathing, simply remain aware of it. This is called passive conscious breathing. As your mind focuses on your breath, you become aware of your inhale and exhale. Then, as you continue your observation over a number of breaths, you may notice a momentary retention of the breath after the inhalation, and possibly a slight suspension after the exhalation. As your mind becomes more fully absorbed in this observation of the breathing process, the character of the breath tends to change involuntarily. In other words, your breath changes simply by your being aware of it.

In this type of passive observation, you do not attempt to regulate any part of the breathing cycle. You simply notice it, allowing whatever effect may be caused by that awareness to happen. To watch the breath without interfering with it is an illuminating experience, but a difficult one. It reflects a high degree of concentration and is, in fact, almost a state of meditation. Often, this state allows many observations and emotions to surface, and can be quite useful.

The remainder of this chapter will focus on active conscious breathing, the deliberate modulation of breathing patterns over a number of breaths.

The Nature of the Breath

Components of the Breathing Cycle

Breathing is a continuous, rhythmic movement that lasts from the moment of your birth until your death. Its rhythm arises from a cycle of interrelated movements that repeats and renews itself constantly over the entire span of each lifetime. Understanding the components of this cycle illuminates the power of this movement and its effect on the integration of body, breath, and mind.

This breathing cycle consists of four components:

- Exhalation — the outward movement of the breath (*bahya*).
- Inhalation — the inward movement of the breath (*abhyantara*).
- Suspension of the breath after exhalation (*bahya kumbhakam*).
- Retention of the breath after inhalation (*antar kumbhakam*).

This process has been separated into these categories for clarity. In reality, however, they are functionally linked, each one affecting the others. The exhalation elicits the inhalation. The suspension and retention are really the terminal points of expiration and inspiration. As in all aspects of yoga, to change one component is automatically to affect the others. Breathing is thus both an integrated and integrating phenomenon.

In learning about the components of the breath it is necessary to adapt all ideal descriptions to the individual, as in the case of practicing asana. The practice of pranayama should also include the concepts of intelligent effort and the recognition of resistances. Without an awareness of these principles, breathing techniques may be ineffective, or even harmful.

The components of the breathing cycle differ in several ways. Each has a specific set of physical movements and physiological characteristics; each elicits a particular psychological response. More importantly, each part has a different role in the removal of impurities, the primary aim of pranayama.

One important note before we look at the components of breathing: Adaptation is the rule. Before deciding on the best pranayama for a student, a good teacher will learn the student's history. It is important to know, for example, whether a student has a history of chest pain, bronchitis, or chronic headaches before teaching any breathing technique. Furthermore, the teacher will need to observe if the student has the necessary prerequisites for a pranayama practice — good posture, a straight spine, and taut abdomen. Once the teacher knows a student's history and present condition, he or she can design the correct sequence of orderly steps (vinyasa krama) for learning an ideal inhalation or exhalation. It may be that before approaching the breath directly, the student needs to work on his or her posture and abdomen. Whatever the circumstance, appropriate adaptation is critical.

Exhalation

In pranayama the main emphasis is on the exhalation because of its use of the lower abdomen. In the ideal exhalation, your breath is fully removed first from your abdomen and then from your chest. You must complete the expiration before the inhalation begins — that is, all the air that can be comfortably expelled from the lungs should be gone. In the ideal inhalation described above, the lower abdomen is not involved at all. However, in reality, most inhalation does use this area, and so is used in the exhalation as well. The lower abdomen initiates the expiration of the breath, and in doing so performs considerable exercise.

As mentioned above, the lower abdominal area, apana, is the main location of impurities in the body. As such, it is considered the seat of disease. You eliminate these impurities with the help of exhalation. Especially when you begin a practice, a great many impurities have already accumulated, so it is important at this point to make good use of the exhalation to eliminate them. Only then can real progress toward personal reintegration accelerate.

Exhalation has a calming, relaxing effect. Normally, in unconscious breathing, the expiration is a passive response of the upper torso to decrease the air pressure in the chest from the last inhalation. No muscle contraction is necessary to accomplish this involuntary action, which is simply a relaxation of the expanded torso. As the area releases, becoming smaller, air is expelled from the lungs.

In the consciously applied technique of pranayama, however, this movement is actively initiated and accentuated by the voluntary use of the abdominal muscles and accessory breathing muscles in the torso. Yet the soothing, relaxing characteristic of the expiration remains. Just as a sigh signifies a release of tension, purposeful emphasis on expiration has a tension-reducing effect.

Inhalation

The inspiration of air into the lungs is an active process, in which you actively expand the chest and straighten the spine. Ideally, the inhalation begins in the chest and progresses to the upper abdominal area. In the most idealized version you keep the lower abdominal area below the navel contracted, not letting it move downward or outward. For all but the most experienced students, however, this type of inhalation results in tension in the neck and abdominal areas, and may cause problems related to the spinal column. The more workable version for all students allows the lower abdomen to become somewhat involved at the end of the inhalation, moving outward slightly.

The inhalation is the active and invigorating portion of the breathing cycle. Even in unconscious breathing, inspiration is accomplished by the active use of muscles. In contrast, the normal unregulated expiration is simply a passive response. Thus, the psychological and physiological effects of a practice emphasizing inhale are of an activating, revitalizing nature. Your energy is enhanced and your mood is uplifted. Such effects are useful before work or any activity demanding physical or mental energy, and can be psychologically helpful in dealing with depression or low self-esteem.

Suspension and Retention

In normal breathing we are not conscious of the end points of our inhalation (retention) or exhalation (suspension). Occasionally we involuntarily retain the breath when lifting a heavy object or gasping in fright, but generally these points where the the breath changes direction are unnoticeable. In pranayama, however, these segments of the breathing cycle are intentionally lengthened to generate various benefits.

Although both retention and suspension involve holding the breath, they differ considerably not only in how they are done, but in their difficulty and function. Retention is a method of extending the inhale. Since the chest is expanded and the spine is straightened during the inhale, retention of the breath holds the muscles in this position, increasing their range of motion and the general flexibility of the torso. Naturally, as the muscles associated with breathing become stronger and more supple, one's respiratory capacity becomes much greater. In addition, this open-chested stance, long associated with assertion and openness, can be helpful in increasing self-confidence.

Suspension — holding the breath after exhaling — is a technique for extending the exhale. The abdominal muscles work in this process and can become noticeably stronger in doing so. This development will enhance the ability to perform effective pranayama, as well as contributing to one's general health.

To learn how to retain and suspend the breath, it is best to begin with suspension. After you exhale, it is impossible to voluntarily hold your breath for any long period. You will automatically gasp for breath after a certain amount of time, a warning that the physiological limit has been reached.

After you inhale, on the other hand, it is possible by sheer will power to voluntarily hold the breath beyond the limits of safety and effectiveness. There is no physiological warning signal, so going beyond your limits can happen inadvertently, causing many problems. Retaining the breath is beneficial when performed correctly, but it is best to begin with suspension and then, after some experience in this and the necessary conditioning of the torso, to progress to retention.

The Relationship Between the Various Components

There is an intricate association between the four components of the breath. In general, this relationship takes the following form:

1. One component influences the other. For example, a very long inhale causes the exhale to become short and fast.

2. One component helps develop the other. For example, retention (holding after the inhale) helps develop the inhale itself.

3. One component disturbs the other. For example, excessive retention can disturb exhalation, shortening it and disrupting its smoothness. Similarly, excessive suspension can disturb the inhalation.

In this perpetual cycle where each segment of the breath affects the others, the resulting process is a balanced and integrated one. Inspiration and expiration mutually create, balance, and support each other. Exhalation removes or destroys, while inhalation creates or acquires.

It is interesting to note that while the actual inhale itself has a definite limit, the hold after it can be extended voluntarily. However, despite exhalation generally being much longer than inhalation, the suspension following it can only be short.

Each breathing component also has a different function in the process of burning impurities. The breath is the support for the internal flame. It is the method by which impurities are moved toward it and carried away from it out of the body. The inhalation moves the flame downward (see figure) toward the impurities in the the lower abdomen, or apana, and burns them.

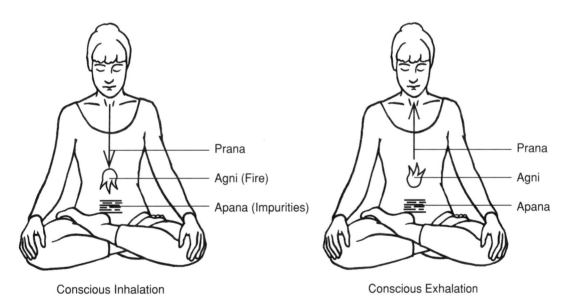

Conscious Inhalation   Conscious Exhalation

During retention this burning continues. On exhalation the burned remnants of the impurities are expelled from the body. During suspension, the remaining dirt is brought upward nearer the flame for more effective burning. (Inversion can be used to accomplish this same action, because when one is upside down, the dirt is pulled downward toward the flame by the force of gravity.)

Once you know the characteristics of these components, their effects, and the techniques for performing them, you have a wide spectrum of tools for designing a personalized pranayama practice. At the same time, the guidance of an experienced teacher is *essential* in learning and practicing this. Depending on the condition of the student and the intended goal, a good teacher will select an appropriate approach. He or she will emphasize certain characteristics or techniques, delay others, orient the practice toward producing a specific psychological effect or developing a certain part of the breath.

The characteristics of the four components of the breathing cycle are summarized below.

No.	Component of breath	Distinct features
1.	EXHALE	• Contraction • Body goes down • Relaxes body
2.	INHALE	• Expansion • Body goes up • Straightens spine • Brings out increased alertness
3.	SUSPENSION AFTER EXHALATION	• Works on stomach • Not possible to suspend breath by "will" beyond limits
4.	RETENTION AFTER INHALATION	• Similar to Inhale • Works more on chest • Possible to hold by "will"

Types of Pranayama

You consciously regulate your breath by changing the duration of one of the four components of the breathing cycle. Because your mind and body are connected, this will transform your state of mind. You can control the duration of all components at the same time, or only one or two of them. The ancient texts emphasize three types of breathing patterns:

• Lengthening the exhalation (*rechaka* pranayama).
• Lengthening the inhalation (*puraka* pranayama).

- Lengthening the suspension or retention of the breath (kumbhaka pranayama).

When the length of the inhalation and exhalation are equal, the technique is called *samavritti* pranayama. "Sama" means equal, and "vritti" means movement. When the inspiration and expiration are not equal, this is called *vishamavritti* pranayama, unequal movement. For example:

- Inhale 8 seconds, exhale 8 seconds is an "equal movement" (samavritti) pranayama.

- Inhale 8 seconds, exhale 16 seconds is an "unequal movement" (vishamavritti) pranayama.

The relationship between the amount of time spent in the various parts of the breathing cycles is called a ratio. The duration of each is written in this order: inhalation, retention, exhalation, suspension. If no retention or suspension is to be stipulated, it may simply be written inhalation: exhalation.

The numbers may reflect actual time, in terms of seconds, or the relationship of one component to the other. Therefore, if we inhale 8 seconds, and exhale 16 seconds without retention or suspension, the ratio is 8:0:16:0 (seconds) or 1:0:2:0.

Inhale: 8 seconds
Retention after the inhale: None
Exhale: 16 seconds
Suspension after the exhale: None

If we then add 8 seconds of retention and 8 seconds of suspension, the ratio become 8:8:16:8, or 1:1:2:1.

The variation in ratios is endless. To select an appropriate one, you must have a thorough knowledge of the characteristics of each component and of the intricate relationship between them, as well as a clear understanding of what comprises a successful pranayama practice. This, we cannot emphasize enough, is where a teacher's role is critical.

Methods of Breathing

People generally breathe through their nostrils, although there are several other methods. The most notable of these is breathing through the mouth. There are also other lesser known techniques that can be beneficial for specific reasons relating to the practice of yoga. Using your fingers to control the flow of air, you may breathe with one nostril half-closed and the other fully closed, or you may inhale and exhale through different nostrils. You can breathe with your tongue curled or folded so that air is sucked in through it, producing a cooling effect; you can also produce the ujjayi sound in the throat. In addition, you may also use certain words to lengthen the exhalation.

No.	Name	Inhale	Exhale	Remarks
1	Anuloma Ujjayi	Throat	Alternate nostrils	
2	Viloma Ujjayi	Left nostril/right nostril (alternate)	Throat	
3	Pratiloma Ujjayi	Throat Left nostril Throat Right nostril	Left nostril Throat Right nostril Throat	1 round consists of 4 breaths
4	Sitali	Mouth with folded tongue	Throat or one nostril	
5	Sitkari	Mouth with tongue flat between slightly opened teeth	Throat or one nostril	
6	Nadi Shodana	Left nostril Right nostril	Right nostril Left nostril	1 round consists of 2 breaths
7	Surya Bhedana	Right nostril	Left nostril	
8	Chandra Bhedana	Left nostril	Right nostril	
9*	Kapala Bhati	Both nostrils stomach forward	Both nostrils stomach in	This is fast abdominal breathing
10*	Bhastrika	Left nostril Right nostril	Left nostril Right nostril	This is fast abdominal breathing
11	Murcha	Deep	Long	Extended exhale. This is a pranayama with emphasis on exhale.
12	Plavini	Quick inhale and long hold after inhale	FREE	Emphasis is on holding after inhale.

* These are classified under kriyas.

Ancient yogis gave a great deal of attention to the various aspects of breathing and to the effects of such techniques. They found that the correct use of certain patterns was helpful in correcting bodily imbalances, enhancing existing strengths and restoring health. Several of these were incorporated into the practice of pranayama. As a matter of interest, the chart on the preceding page shows a number of these possibilities. Further elaboration is beyond the scope of this text, whose aim is to present the main essence of pranayama rather than to describe its less central aspects.

The Qualities of Correct Pranayama

Pranayama and asana are both methods of centering and directing prana. Asana plays two key roles in your preparation for pranayama. First, it prepares the mind by giving it practice in focusing. If you cannot focus on a gross activity like raising and lowering your arms, you will have a harder time focusing on something less obvious, like your breath. Second, it prepares the body. To practice pranayama effectively you need to be in a comfortable position so that your body doesn't disturb your mind as it links itself to your breathing.

Given that the breath can influence the body and mind, the process of doing this should be gradual and subtle so as not to jolt the body and upset the mind, and thereby create resistance. Indeed, you should not even be able to notice the change while it is occurring; rather, you should be able to discern the effects of the practice only after you complete it. With practice, you will also notice changes in your daily life and consciousness.

According to the *Yoga Sutras*, correct asana practice ultimately leads a student to become less disturbed by pairs of opposites or extremes. In asana this is accomplished by achieving the qualities of sthira and sukha, relating to strength and suppleness. In pranayama the aim is the removal of impurities to improve the state of the mind, so that it can become clear and focused. The qualities necessary for this effect are called *dirga* and *sukshma*.

Dirga is translated as "long and steady," a definition which has several levels of meaning. On one level, dirga refers to the length and steadiness of your practice, represented in terms of the duration and regularity of your practice over days, weeks, months and years. Dirga also refers to the manner in which the mind is focused during a practice — how long and how steadily one maintains an introspective stance. If a mantra is used as part of the practice, dirga applies to how long one remains focused on the divinity of that mantra.

Sukshma is defined as "smooth and subtle," and also is understood in various ways. In addition to this usual meaning, it also signifies "inside" or "internal." The more subtle the breath, the more easily you can travel inward, and the higher the quality of your reflection. The smoothness of your breath indicates sustained concentration. If you use a mantra in your pranayama, sukshma represents how smoothly you receive the divinity of the mantra into yourself.

Dirga and sukshma have a dynamic association, each affecting the other. The duration of your practice can affect its smoothness. If you are able to maintain sukshma over a period of time, there will be dirga. The two are inseparable and central to the practice of pranayama. No matter what ratio or technique you chose, your breath should be long and steady (dirga), and smooth and subtle (sukshma).

Attaining the Qualities of Correct Pranayama

Just as the *Yoga Sutras* describes using intelligent effort (prayatna), recognition and reduction of resistance (shaitilya), breath (ananta), and aim (samapatti) to accomplish strength and flexibility, it also presents three essential factors necessary for achieving dirga and sukshma. These are *desha, kala* and *samkhya.* Along with the components of the breathing cycle and their interrelationship, these elements form the basis for a sound pranayama practice.

Desha: Where the Mind is "Placed."

Desha, translated as "place," refers to the role of the mind in pranayama. The sutra places it first in the list of essentials for practice, signifying that it is the most important of them. In this usage, "place" pertains not to a physical area, but to the the mental place where the mind is focused.

It is vital in pranayama that the object of concentration be such that harmony between the mind and the breath is assured. If your mind and breath are at cross purposes, as when your attention wanders to anticipated exciting activities or emotional events of the past, you cannot focus your mind, which is the main aim of the practice. The object of concentration may be external or internal, gross or subtle; for instance, it may by the throat or nostril sound, a chakra or a mantra which represents God. Since mantra is an important aspect of pranayama, before going on to talk about kala and samkhya, we will take a look at the role of mantra.

The role of mantra: The ancient texts defined pranayama as the breath and mind linked to God by means of a mantra. Traditionally, pranayama done with mantra is considered the most significant aspect of all yogic practice and, in the strictest sense, breathing techniques without mantra may not truly be considered pranayama. A mantra is a sound, word or group of words that represents a particular aspect or name of God. It can be recited aloud, with lip movement, or mentally, while the mind focuses on God. Because the actual recitation of the mantra takes a specific amount of time to complete, its structure automatically controls the length of inhalation, retention, exhalation, and suspension. The time during which the mind dwells on God is extended by increasing the number of cycles, or full breaths.

Given the extremely powerful nature of mantra, it is important to practice only with an appropriate one, presented by a teacher who has knowledge of and experience with the mantra, as well as an acute awareness of the student's needs and characteristics. An unsuitable mantra can cause problems that will hinder the student's overall yogic practice and general well-being. Access to such teachers is not always possible, so it is fortunate that pranayama without mantra also provides significant benefits.

The focused visualization of God during pranayama can yield positive results, while an accurate but mechanical repetition of a ratio can become sterile, dull, and unproductive. Your intention and concentration are the keys to progress. The traditional description of the breathing is as follows: On the inhalation, we invite God inside; as we retain the breath we pray to God, invoking God to remain within us; on the exhale we pray that God remove our impurities; and during suspension, we surrender ourselves at the feet of God. We repeat this cycle long enough to become immersed in the link with God. With this sustained focus, pranayama becomes vibrant, active, and meaningful; it is meditation.

Kala: Time and Ratio

Kala, meaning "time," is listed next in the sutras as a necessary element of pranayama. This refers to the duration of the inhalation, exhalation, retention, and suspension. It is the basis for determining whether the pranayama is of equal ratio (samavritti) or unequal ratio (vishamavritti). Different durations of the four components cause different results, so the purpose of the practice will dictate how this factor is used.

Samkhya: The Number of Breaths

The third essential in the practice of pranayama is samkhya, meaning "number." It refers to the number of breaths to be included in a given practice and, consequently, to the total amount of time spent doing it. Because pranayama involves changing the pattern of breathing, the length of this period is important. It must be long enough to effect a change, but short enough to be feasible and comfortable.

Desha, kala and samkhya are connected among themselves, and are also related to the components of the breathing cycle. All must be considered in the design of a safe and productive pranayama practice.

Physical Prerequisites for Practice

As we have mentioned before, if your mind is to focus exclusively on the object of its concentration, your body must be comfortable and steady so as not to cause any distraction. The posture in which you can be steady and comfortable will vary, depending on the purpose of your practice. This can be anything from a therapeutic use, such as helping insomnia, to meditation using mantra.

If the purpose is a therapeutic one, there are few prerequisites. The orientation in this case is on the breathing, not the posture, which should simply be as comfortable as possible. The teacher must determine what position is most suitable and comfortable given the limitations and specific situation of the students. For example, in treating sleeplessness the appropriate posture might be lying in bed, and the time of practice just before going to sleep.

On the other hand, if the purpose relates to meditation, ancient yoga texts list several prerequisites for the correct practice of pranayama:

- The physical ability to sit firmly and comfortably in a suitable posture for an extended period of time.
- Proper preparation for breathing.
- Control of the senses, in order to focus the mind and remain still in a seated posture for a period of time.
- The proper type of food consumed in the correct quantities, i.e., light food in moderate amounts.
- Most important, the guidance of a good teacher, i.e., one with knowledge and experience in pranayama practice and mantra, as well as a familiarity with the student and his or her needs and abilities. The word *guru* is derived from the roots "gu" meaning "darkness" and "ru" meaning "removal," and can also mean "that which is very heavy." The teacher has the weighty position of removing darkness.

We accomplish the first two prerequisites by a well-designed asana practice. The main criteria for the right posture is that it let the body be stable and comfortable so that it will not disturb the quality of the breath. The *Yoga Sutras* does not stipulate any specific posture, but simply states that a student should work on pranayama *after* he or she masters a posture. Pranayama may be done standing, lying down, or seated on the floor or in a chair. The common factor in all these is a certain straightness of the spine that will keep the chest and abdomen free and relaxed for breathing.

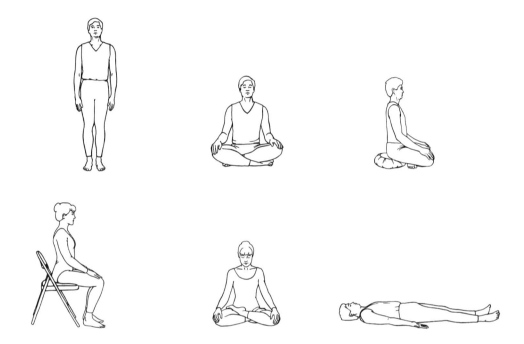

A standing posture offers little stability and comfort, and is generally not used for regular pranayama practice. The exception is its use during the daily ritual of Prayer to the Sun in the morning. Lying down provides the maximum stability, but also too much comfort which is not conducive to focusing the mind. In this position the student's attention may wander or he or she may even fall asleep. Consequently, this posture is used primarily for therapeutic purposes.

The seated posture provides the greatest level of stability and comfort. It is generally possible to remain in a seated position for a prolonged period; therefore it is the posture recommended in the ancient texts for the practice of pranayama. Although the cross-legged seated position is most often associated with pranayama, it is not the most useful posture if you are uncomfortable in it. Of primary importance in selecting the posture is that it not produce tension. In such cases, sitting on a chair or stool is the better choice.

Some General Guidelines for Pranayama Practice

1. In practicing pranayama, the main priority is to establish a breathing pattern that is long and smooth. A short, irregular, and choppy breathing pattern indicates an imbalanced body and mind. If you have this imbalance, you will need to re-evaluate the technique, and modify some or all of its physical and mental characteristics.

2. The results of the practice should be positive. Pranayama is considered the highest of all tapas (methods of "cooking," or removing, impurities). Therefore, the prerequisites and preparation for practice are akin to the preparation of the fire and vessel used in cooking. The various components of breath, place, time, and number are like the ingredients, and must be chosen carefully.

    Dirga and sukshma may be said to represent the quality of the food, while pranayama is the actual cooking process. Just as the proof of good cooking is food that gives energy and removes waste products, the proof of successful pranayama is that it removes mental impurities and focuses the mind. It is therefore advisable to spend some time reflecting on the quality of one's practice, so that the necessary adjustments may be made to improve its results.

3. The breathing ratio must be such that it lets you practice deeply for the entire duration you have planned. In other words, your exhale should not be so long that you need to gasp as you inhale. A breathing cycle with a higher ratio or longer duration does not represent a better practice. Progress is not determined by the length of any breathing component or by increasing your respiratory volume or breathing capacity (although these, too, will improve), but by the resulting clarity of your mind. Just as strength and flexibility in asana practice are related and affect each other greatly, so too are length and smoothness of the breath. Therefore, a balance between the two must be your goal.

4. Investigate the nature of your body, breath, and mind each time before you practice. Various factors affect your breathing ability, and these limits will change constantly. One day's practice may need to be quite different from the last. For example, a heavy

meal late at night may result in shorter breath the following morning. Your practice must be adapted to accommodate for that change, in order for the practice itself to be effective.

It is often a part of human nature to push ourselves to break records, to do as well as we've previously done, and to push ourselves beyond what is truly appropriate at the moment. You can force the body beyond its limits by will power alone, but it is not possible to do so with the breath. Trying to do so will only result in unpleasant and negative effects.

5. Sometimes during the practice of pranayama, certain associations, emotions, or thoughts will arise. If this happens, shift your attention away from the distracting thought to the length or sound of the breath, to a mantra, or to any aspect that will allow you to keep your mind focused. If necessary, you may concentrate on a certain part of the body if that is helpful, and then later direct your focus back to the quality of your breath. It is always easier to begin with the gross and move to the subtle. In this case, the important thing is to direct your attention away from the distraction and eventually back to your breath.

6. In beginning and ending pranayama practice, it is important to follow the appropriate steps, or vinyasa krama, and gradually increase or decrease the length of your breathing cycle back to its normal rate. For example, after practicing pranayama with bandhas, do simple breathing with a ratio of 1:0:2:0 at 6:0:12:0 seconds for several breaths before ending your practice. It is also advisable to rest and reflect on your practice, in order to become aware of any changes that might make your next practice more effective.

To briefly summarize:

- Evaluate your body, breath, and mind before you practice.
- Determine the purpose of your practice.
- Choose the correct type of pranayama and posture for it.
- Choose the appropriate ratio for this practice.
- Start with shorter breathing cycles, and gradually work toward lengthening them. Begin with simpler ratios and advance toward more complex ones over a period of time.
- End the practice gradually.
- Rest and reflect when you are done.

Notes of Caution

The proper practice of pranayama will certainly lead you to an increased sense of well-being and health. However, the incorrect application of breathing techniques can cause problems. The guidance of a good teacher is the best safeguard against these risks, but evaluation and awareness of your own reactions and feelings must be a continuing part of every practice.

The effects of pranayama can be both physical and psychological. During a practice, suppressed emotions or memories as well as unpleasant associations and fears may surface. This can lead to reactions such as crying or depression. A good teacher will know something about the student's psychological state before teaching pranayama. Indeed, this is part of the rationale for starting a yoga practice with asana rather than pranayama. Asana is not only less apt to produce these effects; it allows a teacher to observe the student for a period of time, learning more about his or her physical and mental characteristics before beginning pranayama training.

Ayurvedic texts list the breath as one of the physical urges (*vegas*). These include such actions as sneezing, coughing, urination, and so on. Suppression of these natural urges produces unfavorable reactions in the body. Also, practicing pranayama after running or any activity strenuous enough to change one's breathing can result in chest pain, and is therefore not advised. Instead, you must always allow your breathing cycle to return to normal for some time before gradually beginning your pranayama practice. Otherwise, some of the problems that can be caused by incorrect practice are tension, hiccups, bronchial disorders, and pain in the eyes.

The greatest risk is pushing past your limits. This generally takes the form of overextending the length of one of the breathing components. The most hazardous of these is an overly long retention, or holding too long after the inhalation. The prolonged holding beyond one's limits can aggravate certain underlying conditions, and may result in tremor, pain, or even hernia. Although retention may be useful for a strong, healthy person with a poor self-image, it can be harmful for those suffering from heart disease, neck problems, or insomnia. Additional reactions to this and other incorrect practices can be a tightening of the body, breathing difficulties, and heart palpitations.

Clearly such problems should never be the result of a pranayama practice. It is the responsibility of the teacher to adapt the posture, breathing technique, and ratio to avoid risks and to provide a productive and enjoyable course.

Bandhas

The role of bandhas in pranayama is to facilitate the burning, or purification process, in which impurities are burned and removed from the system. Their purpose is to control the location of these impurities, to direct the flame that burns them, and to efficiently channel the air that fuels the flame and expels the dirt out of the body. Bandhas are muscular contractions that tighten certain parts of the torso to direct the prana accurately toward the flame, to move the dirt in the apana nearer to the fire and to efficiently remove the remnants of the burned impurities during exhalation. Bandha means "to bind, seal or lock." The actions seal off certain areas, directing the flow of prana or impurities along the most useful path.

In the diagram below, note the location of prana, centered in the upper chest at the top of the torso. Apana, considered the site where dirt resides

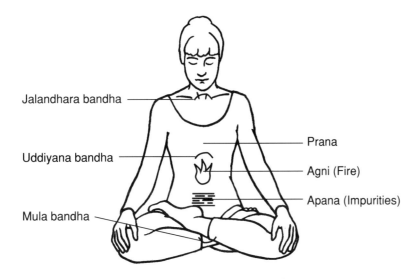

and therefore the seat of disease, lies at the very bottom of the torso. When the torso is sealed at both ends, the prana and apana are linked, so that you enhance the burning of impurities. You can use another bandha to actually move the apana upward nearer the flame; you can also direct the flame, or agni, toward the apana by an accurately directed inhalation. During the bandhas, the torso is essentially sealed, so that the combustion process can progress more efficiently.

A student needs instruction from a knowledgeable and experienced teacher to practice the bandhas. This is due to the sophisticated nature of learning bandhas, and the danger of their misuse. If you feel a strong longing to learn the bandhas, you should seek out a worthy teacher to instruct you.

While the bandhas remove impurities more than pranayama alone, you can accomplish the same intensity of purification by other means, such as sound, without the risk of problems caused by their incorrect use.

The Use of Sound in Pranayama

Sound involves breathing, and is therefore a natural adjunct to the purification process of pranayama. Chanting is extremely powerful in bringing about change and good health. It focuses the mind, elicits internal awareness, and regulates the breath.

You produce sound as you expel air. You can substitute sound for a long exhalation during pranayama. The quality of the sound, its smoothness, volume, and length are indications of the quality of the exhale. You can only make a long smooth sound if you are exhaling correctly. You can even use sound to regulate the breathing cycle, since the number of words or syllables and the loudness of a chant determines the length of the exhale.

Sound produces a different vibration from that of normal breathing. Various sounds produce their own unique vibrations depending on which parts of the body they use. This is why sound is effective in focusing your mind. In focusing on these sensations, you may experience a new awareness of your diaphragm or abdominal area.

In asana there can be tension in the systems, particularly when you are performing difficult postures where your attention is on the form. In chanting and pranayama, however, the focus is much more internal and more subtle.

There are several physical effects of sound. Chanting is considered to be a good exercise for the body and breath, and is beneficial in maintaining optimum health. It can serve as a good preparation or substitute for the bandhas, because it brings about a contraction in the lower abdomen, and is a safer approach.

Pranayama serves to cleanse the body, breath, and mind of the impurities that cloud clarity of vision. It is a powerful and easily accessible tool that, when practiced correctly and regularly, will greatly advance your progress toward personal reintegration.

7

MEDITATION

The Process of Meditation

The ultimate goal of personal reintegration is to see clearly and stay
integrated. It is a simple concept and, in the strictest sense, involves only one
thing: the instrument of perception, our mind. However, the path toward this
goal involves the integrated preparation of our attitudes, senses, body, and
breath for this apparently simple, but all-important function. Once these
aspects are balanced and functioning optimally, we can proceed to the matter
of seeing. Meditation, then, is about this process of perception or reflection.

Most commonly, the Sanskrit word dhyana is translated as "meditation."
"Dhyana" derives from the root *dhyai chintayam*. This means "to think or
reflect." It is also understood as the state of samadhi, the culmination of
that reflection. Therefore, meditation can be viewed both as a technique
and a result.

The aim of meditation is to understand what we did not formerly
understand, to see what we have not previously seen, and to be where we
have never been in relation to an object or subject. Meditation is the
unfolding of what is best for each person, and its results can be measured by
the benefits to an individual's self and life. Meditation is discovery.

The process or state of meditation always involves three entities: the
Perceiver, the object or question, and the mind. As discussed in the first
chapter, the Perceiver never changes. It has the innate ability to see clearly,
and is not affected by the three gunas, or characteristics, that comprise
everything else around it.

The object or subject of investigation can be anything that is voluntarily
selected. It can be an external or internal object, or an intellectual inquiry.

For example, it can be a visual symbol, a series of words or sounds, understanding a specific asana, solving a financial dilemma, communicating with God, and so on. The point is that it must be clearly and voluntarily selected. Finally, the mind must be clear and ready to focus on the question, so that the Perceiver may have an unhindered view of it.

Meditation: Dharana, Dhyana and Samadhi

The journey toward clarity is a progressive one, involving a series of discrete but sequential steps. Initially, the mind must be in a state where there is no fluctuation in one's attention, and it must be able to focus on a single object. At this point, having selected an object or question of choice, one links the mind with it. This focusing of the mind on a specific object is called dharana.

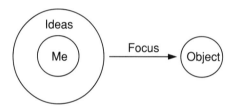

Once this link has been established, the next step, dhyana, becomes possible. In dhyana, the mind continues its communication with, and investigation of, the object. There is interaction — a mental question and answer process — between the mind and the object. The term dhyana is usually translated as "meditation."

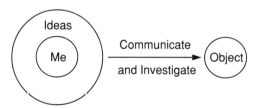

As this interactive process of one-pointed investigation continues, the mind becomes increasingly involved in the object, and ascends to a higher state where it sees what it has not previously seen. Eventually it is totally absorbed in the object. All other thoughts, feelings, mental entities, distractions or perceptions — including the feeling of "I" — temporarily dissolve. At this moment, the object is seen as it truly is, without coloration or distortion of any kind. This state is known as samadhi, and is the state of yoga. The definition of yoga is related to this state (I:2).

When you are totally absorbed in something, you see and understand it as never before. You have a sense of profound discovery. This state of samadhi can occur anywhere, whether you intend it to happen or not, because it is about seeing clearly what you have not seen before.

These three steps must occur in the above order: dharana leads to dhyana, which culminates in samadhi. However, this process is not bound by time. It is not always necessary to sit down with closed eyes. You may be

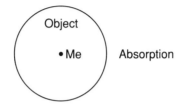

looking at something and, suddenly, what you have not previously understood becomes totally clear to you. It may happen instantaneously, or may happen over a long period of time. It is a temporary state, although its duration may vary. In this final state of yoga, the mind is not affected by the three gunas, impurities are removed, and all objects are perceived clearly. Your actions are then consonant with reality, which is what assures the freedom from suffering.

Meditation is understood in many ways, particularly in the West. According to the *Yoga Sutras*, this is acceptable, since reflection — no matter how primitive or untrained — is still reflection and will lead to a higher state of mind. The *Sutras* further say that one who continues the process ascends to higher and higher states, until finally his or her mind becomes like a telescope that can see any place, any time, and any thing without preparation of any kind. There is no need to deliberately focus, because the mind is like a clear-cut crystal. One simply sees. In this highest state, a person is able to see any subject clearly.

Prerequisites

Having a Clear Question

Meditation is the process of discovery — of moving from one point to another. It therefore entails an examination of some object or question. The aim of the movement must be clear, in order for one to make progress. When there is no aim, or when one's aim remains static and unable to evolve, there is no movement and therefore no meditation. In fact, any mechanical technique that does not result in new knowledge or awareness cannot truly be called meditation. Concentration, relaxation, or visualization may be such techniques, and may be extremely beneficial in improving sleeping habits, and in relieving stress and other related problems. At the same time, they are not yoga.

Leaving Things Behind

The movement toward personal reintegration is a sort of journey. Consequently, it involves leaving things behind. Meditation, like yoga as a whole, is a process of deletion, not addition. When we take a trip, we cannot be both on the platform and on the train. Nor can we travel efficiently if we try to bring everything we have with us. In fact, doing so will ensure that we never reach our destination.

In meditation, what must be left behind are our ideas or preconceived notions about the object of our attention, our inaccurate memories and associations with this object, and all our reactions to it. We must let our ideas, impressions, likes, and dislikes drop from our mind, so that they don't impede clear vision. We may have to let go of some physical things such as certain foods or practices that make the mind unsteady and unable to focus. When this doesn't happen, meditation can become purely a matter of imagination and fantasy, rather than the true discovery it is intended to be. The mind possesses extraordinary powers of creation and imagination that can lead us either into freedom or into bondage.

Reducing Disturbances of the Body, Breath, and Mind

In Chapter 1, the five possible states of mind listed in the *Yoga Sutras* were described. To review, these were:

1. The Agitated Mind: The mind, wanting to be everywhere, actually ends up being nowhere. Prana is diffused and lacks direction. The texts compare the mind in this state to a drunken monkey bitten by a scorpion.
2. The Dull Mind: The mind is dull and heavy. It is present, but at the same time, not present, due to its dullness.
3. The Distracted Mind: There is fluctuation of attention. The mind focuses on the intended object, but then becomes distracted and wanders elsewhere.

4. The Focused State: The mind is focused and able to sustain its attention. Prana moves in one direction. At the same time, the object can trigger associations that may cause some distortion. So, although there is a greater degree of clarity than in the preceding states, accurate and complete perception is not entirely assured.

5. The State of Absorption: This is the clear state in which the mind is so involved in the object that nothing can distract it. It is totally absorbed. Perception is clear, since no memory, imagination, or association hinders one's vision. The object is seen as it is. This state is known as samadhi and the definition of yoga is related to this state (I:2).

Our minds are generally in the first three states, due to certain intrinsic characteristics of the mind, or extrinsic obstacles such as disease, heaviness, fatigue, and so on. These obstacles produce disturbances which don't allow the mind to focus properly. The last two states are the desirable ones in which meditation can take place. Only these two states can truly be considered yoga.

The *Yoga Sutras* (II:53) states that through pranayama the mind becomes fit for focusing. Asana, in turn, readies the body for pranayama. Therefore, these two practices are the usual means for bringing the mind to a focused state. During asana practice, the mind must stay linked to the breath and movement in all postures. Even in difficult postures where your mind will tend to focus mostly on the body, you should keep your attention on your breath.

Indeed, without a clear aim, the capacity to leave behind the impediments to clear vision, and the ability to focus your mind without disturbances, true meditation cannot take place. These preparatory conditions pave the way for the clarity that leads to total personal reintegration.

Stages of Meditation

All travel or movement includes a period of preparation, the stay at one's destination, and finally the return. Likewise, successful meditation involves similar stages. These are classified in the yoga texts as the preparation, the stay, and the return. The three are related, such that poor attention and quality in the one will definitely hinder the quality of the others. In the same way, preparation that is well done will enhance the stages of staying and returning.

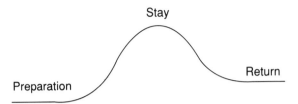

Preparation for meditation is primarily the process of eliminating the obstacles that prevent you from focusing your mind. Pranayama, which is essential to this process, is therefore a part of this stage. Without this stage, we run the risk of simply remaining in the realm of imagination and fantasy, and never approaching our true destination.

To remain in a focused state and be absorbed in the object of meditation is the aim of meditation. The quality of your contact with the object of your attention is, of course, affected by the quality of your preparation.

Finally, there is the return to the normal state of awareness. If the initial preparation has not been adequately done, there can be no return, since there has been no real travel.

These stages represent states of mind in a period of intense focus. They have nothing to do with the object of focus itself, yet they greatly affect how it is perceived. All phases will be present in any successful meditation practice.

Additional Notes on Meditation

Siddhis

Continued focus on any specific object of inquiry through dharana, dhyana, and samadhi over an extended period of time is called *samyama*. This intense and prolonged practice results in a comprehensive knowledge of that object. Extraordinary knowledge and capabilities can be acquired through the practice of samyama. As one continues the practice, one sees more and more deeply. The extraordinary abilities and knowledge that come out of this process are called *siddhis*. In a state of siddhi, what is ordinarily not possible becomes possible. Samyama is a means to this state.

Siddhis are a trap. The person is in danger from his own achievements, from his own successes. The mind becomes unidirectional and yet can still color perception. Siddhis are not extraordinary accomplishments for the person who wants to travel to freedom. Mind is still the master. The ultimate benefit of yoga, which is freedom, can be achieved only if siddhis and their benefits are rejected completely. Remember that siddhis can make you a knowledgable person but not the knower.

Meditation and God

The topic of meditation is often associated with a discussion of God, centering on the question of whether God alone should be the object of meditation, or whether other objects will serve as well. Since yoga deals with the clarifying of one's vision and is not concerned with the actual object of that vision, one might ask why the object should be God rather than some other object.

God is the ideal object of reflection because of the profound influence any object of meditation has upon us. In a sense, we become more and more *like* the object as we begin to perceive and assimilate its characteristics. As God is the highest and most worthy being, it is only logical that God should be the object of meditation. When we are able to do this, we are less ourselves as limited individuals, and more God. The *Yoga Sutras* also cites God as a means of elevating the mind to the state of yoga.

Mantra and Meditation

Mantra is a link to God. A mantra is a series of syllables or words representing God, that is used as an object of meditation. If the student is properly initiated and guided by an experienced teacher, a mantra will provide protection and guidance in the student's practice. God is a guard who protects, a guru who restrains, and a giver who sustains. The connection with the divine through the mantra restrains one who is about to go beyond his or her real limits. This restraint is important, insofar as many of life's problems stem from doing what we should not do. Mantra is also a means of reflection, and increases one's knowledge of oneself.

Symbolism in Meditation

A symbol can also be a means to link oneself to God, and can therefore be useful in meditation. The advantage of symbols is that they transcend cultural barriers, and the associations inherent therein. They are therefore neutral.

Many of the Hindu gods are represented by a letter and a symbol. For example, the Sun god is represented by the letter pronounced *hram*.

Symbols are helpful in understanding ourselves because, since they themselves are neutral, we tend to project what is within us onto them. In this way they become a powerful means of self-reflection.

At the same time, care should be taken in selecting a symbol, for it can influence one's mind and thereby one's actions.

Some General Hints for Meditation

- You must understand the purpose of meditation, and choose the object carefully, for the object will influence your mind and actions.
- You must choose the appropriate model for meditation, based on your needs and nature.
- The techniques that suit the teacher may not necessarily suit the student. Constant assessment and self-study are necessary to assure that your practice is beneficial.
- The Indian tradition of meditation may be unsuitable for Westerners. The practice should be harmonious with one's own culture, tradition, and mental disposition.
- Choose a practice that you can sustain for an extended period, without internal conflict.
- Meditation should not become an escape, or a retreat into any kind of darkness, but rather should lead you into the light of reality. The more we remain in darkness, the less we are willing to face the light. Meditation should be an ever-increasing illumination of reality.

The Importance of the Individual Path

In meditation, as with all the components of yoga, we need to take an integrated look at each person to determine what is appropriate for the individual. It is important to start where you are. This involves an evaluation of your attitudes, inclinations, culture, tradition, beliefs, profession, lifestyle, and so on. You must consider your structural, functional, psychological, and social characteristics. Although it is not always possible, a good teacher who can hold up the mirror of reflection to a student is the most helpful instrument in guiding one's practice.

In the end, meditation *is* what it does for us. If meditation is successful, our minds will be elevated to a higher level and we will become better than we are now. This will be reflected in our actions and, ultimately, will enhance our whole experience of life.

8
YOGA THERAPY

Traditional Yogic Perspectives on Health and Disease

Before we discuss the practical applications of yoga as a therapy, we will outline the traditional yogic view of health, disease, and the restoration of balance. According to this tradition, the universe consists primarily of the following five elements: earth, water, fire, air, and space.

These five elements each contain the three basic gunas we introduced earlier — satva, rajas, and tamas — representing balance, activity, and inertia respectively. As humans, we are also made up of the five elements and the three gunas. Just as what is outside is inside as well, what is in the macrocosm is also in the microcosm. Health is a balance between the two. The science of Ayurveda, the ancient Indian system of medicine, deals with this in great depth.

According to this tradition, the elements are understood to evolve in the following order:

space — air — fire — water — earth

At the same time, each element contains the other, and all of them are interrelated.

According to yogic tradition, the five elements are represented in the body in specific areas along the spine. These areas correspond to what are called the chakras, or centers. Each of these interacts with each of the others. The word chakra literally means "wheel," which symbolizes motion. Chakras themselves represent the motion or changes that continually take place within us. This is only natural, because nothing in us is static, and nothing permanent except change.

There are seven chakras in the body. The first five of these, going from the bottom to the top, correspond to the five elements from earth to space, respectively. The sixth chakra represents the mind and intelligence, and the seventh, the Perceiver (also referred to as *Purusha*). The importance and attention given to the chakras in the yogic tradition is considerable. They represent our emotions, as well as the basic seven notes of music. In each case, they are affected by our state of mind.

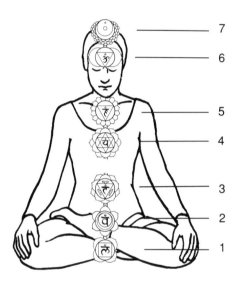

Chakra	Element
1. Muladharam	Solid (Earth)
2. Swadishtanam	Liquid (Water)
3. Manipurakam	Fire
4. Anahatam	Air
5. Visuddhi	Space
6. Ajna	Mind
7. Sahasraram	Perceiver

What is most interesting about the chakras from the perspective of yoga therapy is that a person is healthy when the chakras are in balance and in their proper place. As we noted above, the chakras are not stationary. Structural displacement happens due both to our inactivity and to the wrong kind of activity. Functional disintegration happens due to the lack of personal disciplines (or inappropriate disciplines), as well as to the food we eat, since our food can promote or impede the flow of prana. Psychological disintegration can happen due to emotional disturbances.

When a person is totally integrated, the chakras are in balance and the energy flow is as it should be. The objective of the practice of yoga is to bridge the gap between the actual and the ideal, so that the chakras are brought into their proper places and into balance. We will go on to discuss briefly the role of asana and pranayama in bringing about this state.

The Role of Prana in Health

The ultimate goal of a yoga practice is to ensure that the prana reaches the uppermost chakra, the Sahasraram. We have already discussed the concept of prana (see Chapter 6). To review: Prana is the life force in a human being. It is responsible for the functioning of all the systems, including the mind.

Prana is categorized into ten divisions, each according to its function. These are called the ten *vayus*. Prana flows through subtle channels called *nadis*, along which our life force works in the body. There are fourteen important nadis in the human body. As long as our energy flow in the nadis is as it should be, we experience balance and health. Whenever the flow of energy is obstructed, however, we experience disease. The practice of yoga enables us to remove the impurities that obstruct the flow which, in turn, restores the proper flow of prana.

We remove impurities by the proper use of the fire and air elements in our system. Impurities accumulate in the first place due to food, activity or inactivity, environment, thought processes, and so on. One of the fundamental premises of Ayurveda, for example, is that sickness is due to uncooked food remaining in the system — in other words, that illness is a result of improper digestion and incomplete elimination. The fire element of the human system must therefore be kept at its optimum level for health.

Yoga attempts to remove impurities through proper use of fire and air. These two elements support each other, with air fueling the fire. The following figure represents this process:

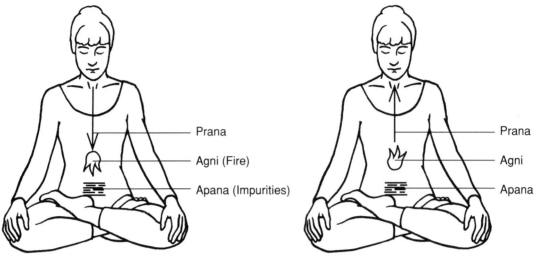

Conscious Inhalation   Conscious Exhalation

During inhalation, we enhance the fire and burn up the impurities. During exhalation, we remove waste from our system. Moreover, different positions of the body change the position of the agni in relation to the impurities. As discussed in the section on Viparita Karani, for example, doing headstand reverses the position of the fire. Likewise, different positions of the body also change the flow of breath and prana.

The Use of Asana to Remove Impurities

In the asana chapter we noted that the primary emphasis in asana should be on the spine. This is because the purpose of asana practice is to align the chakras. This alignment brings about structural integration, which in turn leads to functional and psychological integration.

When we run or do floor exercises, we automatically displace the chakras, due to the fact that we are moving our body without a set direction in regard to the position of agni and the flow of prana. Thus, a yoga practice done without proper consideration of breath and movement may not be very beneficial.

Yoga Therapy: A Therapy Without Medicine, A Surgery Without Tools

In the path toward personal reintegration the first step is to begin to clear away the most destructive obstacles to clear perception. Disease is the most significant of these. When your health is poor, the imbalance and dysfunction inherent in your condition make focusing the mind impossible. Regardless of the technique you use or the amount you practice, progress toward a state of clarity will be greatly hindered, if not entirely blocked.

Disease is, in fact, the indicator or symptom of a disintegrated system. Yoga therapy is the art and science of healing according to yogic principles. It is used as an alternative or adjunct to other kinds of health care. But in the context of one's overall self-improvement, its more significant use is as a method for removing obstacles to clear perception, the first step in personal reintegration.

According to yoga, the body contains impurities from birth, and continues to acquire more through daily existence. This ongoing accumulation occurs because the mind, due to its basic state of misapprehension, is unable to discern between beneficial and harmful actions. It therefore directs our actions incorrectly. This, in turn, causes imbalance in the system. To establish or maintain this balance, the impurities must be continually removed from the system.

The external environment is another factor that affects the human system. Health is the interaction between the system of the body, mind, and breath, on the one hand, and the circumstances in which this system exists, on the other. An imbalance can be caused by either component — the individual or the environment — or by a combination of the two.

There are, of course, variables within each of these components. An individual is characterized by his or her physical structure and function, temperament, mental and emotional nature, and so on. The environment includes not only physical aspects such as the weather, conditions of cleanliness, safety, and comfort, but also the nature of the people involved, the importance of each event, and so on. Both the internal and external factors are constantly shifting.

The ancient teachers and healers considered good health to be a state of integration. Today, the World Health Organization defines health similarly, as a state of physical, mental, and social well-being, and not merely the absence of disease. The early wise men of India went beyond merely describing ill health as an imbalance caused by impurities, and offered, instead, a practical method of restoring balance and good health. In the *Yoga Sutras* (II:29), Patanjali set forth the eight limbs of yoga, which is the practical basis for yoga therapy, or the healing of all aspects of one's being.

These limbs are all expressive of the means by which to bring about a wholistic understanding of health like the one defined by the World Health Organization. The eight limbs are:

1. Yama — social behavior 2. Niyama — personal disciplines	Social Well-being
3. Asana — the body 4. Pranayama — the breath 5. Pratyahara — the senses	Physical Well-being
6. Dharana 7. Dhyana ⎱ the mind 8. Samadhi	Mental Well-being

In turn, the eight limbs are each related to the different aspects of personal reintegration, which are also ways of talking about health.

1. Yama — social behavior	Social Reintegration
2. Asana — the body	Structural Reintegration
3. Niyama — personal disciplines 4. Pranayama — the breath 5. Pratyahara — the senses	Functional Reintegration
6. Dharana 7. Dhyana ⎱ the mind 8. Samadhi	Psychological Reintegration

Total personal reintegration, for which yoga therapy is a starting point, involves all of these processes.

Yoga Therapy: An Individualized Approach

A yoga therapist aims at restoring this balance by understanding the individual, the environment in which the individual is operating, and the interplay between the two, looking for the factors that account for the imbalance. To do this, the therapist observes and learns about all the facets of the person's life and environment, as covered in the eight limbs of yoga. Recognizing that each aspect affects all others, the teacher or therapist must be sensitive to the dynamic relationship among all areas, as he or she searches for the causes of a specific symptom.

The teacher must not only be able to identify the cause, but must then help the student reflect and develop an appropriate program. Simply teaching some postures without reflection or consideration of the breath will not be successful. Rather, the teacher must include all areas of the student's life experience in the treatment. For example, the effect of yoga practice for an asthmatic who continues to smoke and eat heavy, greasy food late at night will at best be palliative, and not curative. A superficial solution to a deeper problem will not work.

Yoga therapy involves no external aids, but uses a person's mind, breath, and body to bring about the balance or harmony of the system that is true good health. Therefore, it is a therapy without medicines and a surgery without tools.

Good health is the natural state of the body when prana (discussed in earlier chapters) flows easily and evenly throughout the body. When its flow to a particular area is blocked, problems will arise at that point. Disease is seen as indicating an obstruction in the optimal flow of prana. Again, the cure is the removal of obstacles that restrict or block this flow, so that good health can be allowed to flourish.

Yoga therapy operates according to the same individualized approach that characterizes all yogic practice. The underlying premise of this system is to treat the whole person, and not just the disease. Therefore, each prescribed course is different. Not only do the areas of treatment differ, but the manner in which they are used vary according to the individual. These programs consider physical exercises, dietary habits, work schedule, family matters, and so on.

Each program considers the patient's current condition, using that as a starting point, and structures the program from that point so as to be safe, feasible, and effective in each individual case. Relaxation techniques and the use of the breath are included to aid healing. Perhaps most important is the fact that the patient, rather than the therapist, does the therapy him- or herself. This places the responsibility on the individual students, keeping them involved in their own progress and motivation, and building confidence in their ability to establish and maintain good health.

In any illness or problem, the therapist usually finds social, structural, functional, and psychological aspects which relate to the cause and cure of the identified symptom. For example, a scoliosis — usually identified as merely a structural problem — will often have associated functional problems, and a myriad of psychological effects as well. In every case, it is absolutely essential to examine as many levels of a person's history as possible, and to include these in the treatment. In this way, each treatment is uniquely fitted to the patient.

The Yogic Approach to Restoration of Balance

To be in balance means that all the elements of one's life function harmoniously. These include: mental attitude, food, hygiene, the body and breath, social interaction, the behavior of the senses, one's state of mind, and so on. To become fully balanced, one must typically address many of these areas. The common means to addressing them involve changes in one's diet and personal disciplines, as well as the practice of reflection or meditation, prayer, asana and pranayama, mantra, and pilgrimage.

Diet

Ideally, food serves several purposes. It provides energy and removes impurities. In addition, food has a significant influence on the mind. We might go so far as to say that food is what you eat, and what can eat you, if you aren't careful. Like God, food accomplishes the three functions of creation, sustenance, and destruction. When your diet does not function to fulfill each of these three roles in a balanced manner, then imbalance and disease will result.

Because food can be a major cause of imbalance, modification of one's diet may be an effective agent in curing the problem. For example, eating gas-forming foods late at night can aggravate symptoms of asthma. Ice cream and cold drinks can also increase the risk of asthma attacks, especially in children.

Each type of food has its own characteristics, and produces specific results when eaten. Certain foods increase the formation of phlegm, and certain spices reduce it. A teacher who is knowledgeable about these effects can be extremely helpful in suggesting a diet that will establish and maintain a balanced system.

Personal Disciplines

Personal habits also have a great effect on one's health. Adherence to different disciplines can shift an imbalanced system into a healthier state. This means the practice of right acts and the cessation of wrong ones. These can range from changing one's eating schedule, bathing habits, or smoking patterns, to revising one's practice of asana, pranayama, and dhyana. For example, many asthmatics experience an improvement if they eat early in the evening or take warm baths rather than cold ones. Giving up smoking will improve many conditions. Some lower back problems are helped by warm showers. In general, personal habits that are appropriate to the individual can increase one's comfort and contentment, allowing the system to move toward equilibrium.

Reflection

Reflecting on the factors that trigger a problem can help determine the actual cause. Since disease stems from a disturbance in the mind, this method of self-discovery can often be very illuminating and useful in treating illness. For example, the asthma patient who tracks down the factors leading to asthma attacks can make changes that prevent them. Many such people have cured this problem by discovering and eliminating a source of tension, such as a stressful job, that provoked the symptoms.

Prayer

An ancient verse states: *Vaidyo narayano Harih* — "God is the greatest healer." A prayer to God is a certain means of restoring balance and harmony in one's system. It is also a method of learning about oneself, and thereby more accurately identifying the cause of a disease.

Asana and Pranayama Practice

Yoga Rahasya, a yoga text, advises, "Use asana to restore balance of the body and pranayama to restore mental balance." As we have seen in our earlier discussion of these topics, these two practices play a central and vital role in the restoration of health.

Pilgrimage

When you find yourself highly disturbed, it is often beneficial to simply step back or even get away from the situation, whether or not it is the actual causal factor. Since change is an element of growth and healing, a different environment may provide a new perspective. It can give you time to re-evaluate your circumstances, a new set of stimuli, or simply a respite from a troublesome situation. There are some cases where the actual environment may be the root of the problem.

Mantra

Mantra can be a powerful agent for balancing the system, depending on the student's reaction to it. Mantra is considered a bridge to God and, when practiced correctly, can bring about considerable change in one's life and health. Abuse of the senses is one of the main causes of imbalance and is, in fact, the source of a great many diseases. Mantra can serve as a protection against temptations which, when acted upon, shift the system out of balance and into a state of ill health. It may be considered a means of catching oneself in time. The importance of an experienced teacher and further details about mantra were discussed earlier.

This list of common approaches used in yoga therapy should serve only as a basic guideline. The effectiveness of treatment depends on the teacher's ability to observe correctly, to understand the essential aspects of a student's nature and problem, to keep an open mind, and to continue to look for solutions that uniquely fit the individual. A good teacher must also be a regular practitioner of yoga, in order that his or her perceptions of both his or her own self, and of the student, remain as clear as possible.

Because a teacher must tailor each program according to the individual student, it is difficult to establish a set of standard procedures for dealing with particular problems, and it is beyond the scope of this book to discuss in detail the procedures by which a trained yoga therapist diagnoses and develops a treatment program for a student.

In general, the teacher must establish a good rapport with the student. This involves approaching each person individually, and coming to know not only the person's physical condition, but also all the other factors we have discussed that play into the development of a health problem. These issues are what will allow the yoga therapist to design a program that will address the specific issues of the particular individual, and to make sure that all parts of the therapy are realistic and comfortable for the student.

Diagnostic Principles of Yoga Therapy

Yoga therapy treats the patient rather than the disease. This means that diagnosis is very important. The disease is examined not as a discrete event occurring separately from the person, but is viewed as part of the individual's personal nature, habits, history, and environment.

A therapist does not merely identify the symptom and prescribe a standard treatment to eliminate it. Instead, he or she recognizes that a specific symptom may reflect different causes in different people, and therefore requires a wide spectrum of treatments, each dependent upon the individual case. This makes diagnosis more complex. It seeks not only to identify symptoms, but also to discover causes. To do this accurately involves obtaining as much pertinent information about the individual and his or her life as possible.

The four principles used for diagnosis are: Observation and inspection (*darshana*, "to see, to look"); Physical examination and palpation (*sparshana*, "to touch, to feel"): Patient history (*prasna*, "to question, to inquire"); and Pulse-taking (*nadi pariksha*, "to look into the whole system through the pulse").

Observation (Darshana)

Visual observation of a person can provide a wealth of information, if done carefully and wisely. It starts at the moment of meeting the student, when he or she is unaware of being observed. When people know they are being watched, their actions change, so the yoga therapist gathers as much information as possible before actually letting the student know that he or she is being watched. Many details in a person's appearance, mannerisms, interaction, and behavior are available and valuable to a careful observer.

One should note all parts of the student's body in terms of structure and manner of functioning: the face, eyes, lips, skin, head and neck, physical build, chest, manner of breathing, abdomen, spine, manner of movement, and so on. One's voice, type of speech, mannerisms, handwriting, degree of comfort in interaction, attitude, and general behavior are all indicators about the student. A skillful teacher is able to glean a lot of information from a few details, and does not need to gather a vast number of facts. This ability makes a session shorter and is easier on both student and teacher.

At some point it usually is necessary either to observe the student doing some simple postures and movements which will demonstrate the problem, or to specifically examine the identified symptoms. This, of course, requires the help and willingness of the student. When testing, it is best to use simple postures that won't intimidate or tire the student, and to get a lot of information from a few postures rather than putting him or her through a long, complicated series of asanas.

If possible, these should be postures in which the student can relax, such as raising the arms while seated, or raising the arms or legs from a lying down position. The purpose of this testing is to determine how the body works, to detect the areas of strength, weakness, or imbalance, and to check one's initial hypothesis about the problem. For example, if a teacher's first idea regarding a student's headaches relates to the neck muscles, a posture that uses the neck will show the strength of the neck, and will indicate whether using the neck muscles makes the headache worse or better. From this information, the teacher can proceed, adapting the testing postures to check other areas, assigning exercises if necessary, and addressing other components of the treatment such as food, lifestyle changes, etc.

Physical Examination (Sparshana)

It is necessary to palpate areas in question to get a sense of their function and condition. The feel of how a movement is executed can provide a lot of information about its biomechanical aspect. Knowing whether certain areas are relaxed or chronically contracted is important, and a sense of a person's muscular development and structural imbalances often can only be learned from this method. The ability to do this well — to know what to look for and how to obtain information without making the student feel discomfort on any level — is an art that requires great sensitivity and careful practice.

It is also often advisable to have students point to the places on their own bodies that they perceive as troublesome, for these may vary considerably from what the teacher observes externally.

Inquiry (Prashna)

This involves questioning the patient about the chief complaint, obtaining as much general information as possible about lifestyle, health history, present state of health and so forth. Questioning is an art in which the patient must be made to feel at ease and willing to reveal personal information in an accurate manner. A patient who feels comfortable with the teacher will offer much information from which the teacher can later select what is relevant to the case. Every new piece of information can be useful in creating a larger picture of the student's disease and its origin.

Pulse-taking (Nadi pariksha)

Nadi pariksha is the examination of the pulse to determine a student's state of health. The pulse is an important indicator of many things, and can be used before and after certain movements or breathing techniques to determine the student's effort, stamina, emotional reactions, and so on. In the example of headaches discussed above, the therapist might take the pulse before and after the asana, in order to determine whether this type of exercise would be appropriate or too much for the student. Noticing the heart rate after walking up stairs or while talking during exercise is also a good indicator of a person's stamina.

The pulse reflects both physical and emotional characteristics, and changes in it related to certain activities or situations reveal a great deal about a student's reactions. Irregularity or rapid increase of the pulse is a signal that the body is pushing its physical or emotional limits. The ability to use the pulse diagnostically is extremely valuable, but involves a great deal of knowledge, skill and experience.

General Guidelines in Practicing Yoga Therapy

Because a teacher needs to tailor each program to the individual student, it is difficult to establish a set of standard procedures for dealing with problems. We offer the following suggestions as a framework from which to begin in assessing and treating a student's problems. We divide these suggestions into two areas: 1) the teacher's personal responsibilities and related ethical concerns of treatment and 2) practical methods of approaching problems according to the principles of yoga therapy.

Responsibilities of the Teacher/Therapist

1. Establish a good rapport with the student. This is perhaps the single most helpful aspect in the treatment of any student with any type of problem. When the relationship between teacher and student is positive, the student will willingly respond to questions, usually adding more information on his or her own. He or she will be more relaxed both in being examined and in following instructions so that both procedures will be easier and more accurate.

The effect of this rapport is so strong that sometimes a good relationship with a teacher who is not technically knowledgable about the problem at hand can still bring about healing. A positive bond or experience created between the two people may allow nature to heal the body. In addition, such a rapport makes the sessions more pleasant for both persons, and students become confident, relaxed, and willing to carry out their programs more responsibly.

Each human being possesses unique emotions, prejudices and experiences. Beyond that, any student with a disease or painful symptom is also experiencing some sort of disturbance even before coming to meet a new teacher. This is further exacerbated by the ordeal of going through an examination, answering personal questions, and going through all the other trials associated with medical treatment.

Many students view yoga therapy as mysterious, or even slightly suspect. Often they come to yoga after having experienced repeated failure in other treatment modalities, and are mistrustful, fearful, or angry. At times they expect more than the teacher can give them. But all of them, in seeking help, place in the teacher's hands their most valuable possession — their health. Each teacher must remain ever aware of the responsibility inherent in this situation.

The ability to make students feel at ease and have confidence in the teacher is the art of yoga therapy. Without a relationship in which the teacher is sensitively attuned to the student's nature and reactions, no amount of knowledge or skill will produce the desired results. The looks, mannerisms, and attitudes of the therapist can have an immediate and strong effect on a sick or uncomfortable student. Such people have an uncanny instinct for sensing hostility, disinterest, or disapproval. In some unfortunate cases, a teacher reminds a student of someone else from a past unpleasant encounter or relationship.

There is no standard method for creating a rapport. It can depend, in part, on the nature of the two personalities and their interaction. It is a delicate skill that develops with experience over time, and it is primarily a matter of sensitivity: the ability to clearly perceive another person, and to respond correctly to those perceptions. The teacher's personal yoga practice and work at self-transformation is the best way of accomplishing this, and is a necessary part of any responsible teacher's job. As one progresses toward personal reintegration, all aspects of oneself are improved. In terms of teaching, a yoga teacher with the capacity for friendliness, understanding, and the dignity of quiet confidence will be successful in establishing the rapport with students that is vital to successful therapy.

2. Approach each person individually. The treatment of the whole person rather than the disease is central to yoga therapy. It is certainly important to be knowledgeable about the problems or diseases one encounters and to have general guidelines for treating them. For example, a teacher should understand that lying-down postures are not indicated in the initial stages for people with breathing difficulties, that leg lifts are not advised for treating acute back problems, and so on. But it is as critical to respect the individual as it is to respect the guidelines. A person suffering from an illness quite often knows more about it than any one else.

Moreover, rarely does a student have just one isolated problem. Any health disturbance usually has associated conditions, and the patient's knowledge and description of these can be invaluable in creating a comprehensive picture of the system. This integrated approach of seeing and using all aspects of a person is the core of yoga itself, and of its application in therapeutic situations.

3. Make sure all parts of the therapy are comfortable for students. The concept of *ahimsa*, or non-violence, should be practiced at all times. Both the process of evaluation and the assigned course should inflict no discomfort on the student. It is important that the student enjoy his or her program enough to continue doing it on his or her own, and also that the results are positive.

Pain is definitely a part of many illnesses, and cannot be avoided in some instances, but the treatment itself should never increase it. In many cases, highly motivated students will tend to overwork and hurt themselves in doing so. It is the responsibility of the teacher to instruct the student in becoming sensitive to pain as an indicator of limitation and a hindrance to healing.

4. Be realistic and practical in terms of goals and treatment. In dealing with a single student's problem, a teacher is indirectly also dealing with the family, all the other people who regularly impact his or her life, the person's financial and social circumstances, and all the other practical aspects that comprise daily living. Whenever some aspect of the treatment involves others or is difficult to enforce, a teacher must make an effort to understand the student's personality and life situation enough to decide whether or not it is even a possibility.

If dietary changes are to be a major component of a person's treatment, it is necessary to know if the spouse does all the cooking, whether or not he or she is able or willing to make the changes, and so on. If the change is not feasible, or if instituting it will cause a great deal of stress, another approach to the problem must be found. Likewise, if a change of scene is advisable, a teacher must determine whether this is a realistic possibility.

It may become helpful to see other family members to solicit their support. In some cases, such as a woman's having problems conceiving or an individual's having certain emotional problems, it may be necessary to treat another family member as well as the student.

Sensitivity to these issues must extend to even more subtle areas. A student's mental attitude, concern with social status, age, and a myriad other psychological components will effect his or her reaction to prescribed treatment. An obese, shy loner may have such resistance to attending a group class that he or she may reject the entire program, even if the class is only a small part of it. A wealthy person who needs an herb that grows in the back yard might never consider picking it there, but will be pleased to pay considerable money for the same thing in a bottle purchased from a pharmacist. A good teacher will be able to sense whether an action will feel appropriate, and thus possible, to a student. This level of discrimination on the part of a teacher is the result of careful observation, much experience, and an ongoing personal practice of his or her own.

Practical Guidelines for Yoga Therapy

1. Collect general information in the first visit. This involves all the principles discussed earlier. In this phase, it is advisable to obtain as much information as possible given the restrictions of time and the student's willingness. One should take a patient history which includes, in part, the following:

- Age
- Occupation
- Family physician
- Description of chief complaint, or present illness.
- Past medical history of student and family.
- Present medication and dosages, and current treatment, if any, used for the identified problem. (It is necessary to know the side effects of medication being used, for these will affect any observations the teacher makes.)
- Personal lifestyle habits such as diet, exercise, stress, etc.
- Present physical condition (strength, flexibility, endurance) and personality characteristics. (This information may be partly obtained verbally and partly by physical examination or inference.)
- Technical reports from other sources, if the student has brought them. A teacher should know how to read and understand the basic types of technical reports about musculoskeletal injuries, blood pressure, etc., because such reports can often disclose things that are contraindicated for that condition. This will help in designing the course.

2. Keep an open mind. As you obtain information, observe details, and begin to see patterns, it is tempting to quickly formulate a single hypothesis and immediately proceed to designing a course based on it. When this happens, you may miss valuable information and waste time pursuing an ineffective course. Even though you may have experienced a similar case in the past, individuals vary greatly, symptoms can reflect very different causes and, therefore, the methods of healing them also vary.

As you develop theories, check them from another angle to see if you are perceiving correctly. Observe everything you can without fitting the details into a preconceived solution. Once you have all the data, you will be better prepared to design the optimal therapeutic program.

3. Start the course at the level of the student's present condition.
Earlier we discussed the concept of vinyasa krama — using intelligent and appropriate steps to work toward a goal. Its use in yoga therapy is even more critical than in normal asana practice, because when an injury or problem already exists, the potential for further damage is much higher than in a strong and healthy person.

In determining where to start you need to recognize the difference between the healing phase and the strengthening phase of therapy. In the acute phase of an injury or illness, when the system is noticeably weakened, you must orient the practice only toward recovery. You must address the specific problem so that the system can be stabilized. In this phase the major portion of the student's attention should focus on recovering from the most noticeable problem — the system should be mobilized to relieve the immediate symptoms.

Once the acute problem has been stabilized, the student is ready for a more generalized approach — a strengthening of the whole system or its weaker parts to prevent further dysfunction. In this preventive phase, the program is usually more active, but is still modified to accommodate the results of the acute period. Clearly, a teacher must be extremely sensitive as to when to begin this sort of work, how much the student can safely and effectively do and the effects and progress in each session. Even though it may be obvious that a certain area of a student's body needs strengthening in order to prevent recurrence of the problem, addressing that area when the student is not ready can cause further injury and will be harmful rather than helpful.

4. Take into account the characteristics and nature of the student.
It is always tempting to duplicate a program or approach that has been successful in a similar condition. Yet each person's unique traits make this shortcut an incomplete assessment, and one that may easily leave out important factors that require entirely different treatment. Not only do students differ among themselves, but each one changes constantly. Areas of resistance, the amount of effort, and appropriate goals change as well. A successful course involves continual observation and adaptation.

5. Determine the area of highest priority for treatment. In some cases, it may be necessary to reduce certain symptoms before anything useful can be done about the root cause of the problem. At other times it may be more fruitful to attend to the basic problem, rather than the symptoms the student has presented.

6. Design a course for this immediate objective.

7. Make sure the student can do the course. Lead the student through the entire course, explaining the details of the breathing or movement, clarifying any diagrams you may be providing. It is ideal to do this without actually demonstrating when dealing with adults, because they will attempt to duplicate exactly what you do, whether or not it is appropriate for their body and/or condition.

There are, of course, occasions — particularly involving complex movements or positions — when showing a movement in a general way is the easiest way to help a student learn. Children may often have difficulty understanding verbal instructions; a demonstration is then a better teaching method.

As you initially guide the student through the course, notice any areas that make him or her uncomfortable or produce tension or unwillingness. Change these so that the course is a pleasant experience.

8. Make each segment manageable. It is extremely important for the student to feel comfortable with a practice. Present the overall therapeutic course in smaller installments so that the assigned practice taught in each session is easily manageable for the student to do on his or her own. Then, during the following session, you may add new things or change portions of the previous practice depending on the student's response and progress. Sometimes the same course may need to be repeated for an extended period; sometimes an entirely new one is necessary.

Specific Applications of Yoga Therapy: Two Sample Case Studies

The following two cases involve two men with similar complaints and some shared characteristics. You will note that the difference in their occupations makes their therapeutic requirements quite different.

Case 1

Age: 45 years
Complaint: Essential hypertension for the past five years
Habits: Moderate, clean, wholesome lifestyle
Family: Married, two children
Occupation: Production shop executive
Height: 5'8"
Weight: 133 pounds
Medication for condition: Yes

Case 2

Age: 44 years
Complaint: Essential hypertension for the past four years
Habits: Moderate, clean, wholesome lifestyle
Family: Married, two children
Occupation: Finance executive
Height: 5'8"
Weight: 188 pounds
Medication for condition: Yes

The production shop executive is under constant stress at his job. He works on the production floor and is on his feet and in motion during most of the day. He is lean and gets plenty of exercise.

In contrast, the finance executive has a secure position in a successful company and experiences little tension at work. He is seated all day, getting no exercise, and is overweight. He needs more exercise, as is reflected in his program. In addition, he was advised to reduce his food intake in order to lose weight.

Case 1
Production Executive — Fourth Lesson — Evening Practice

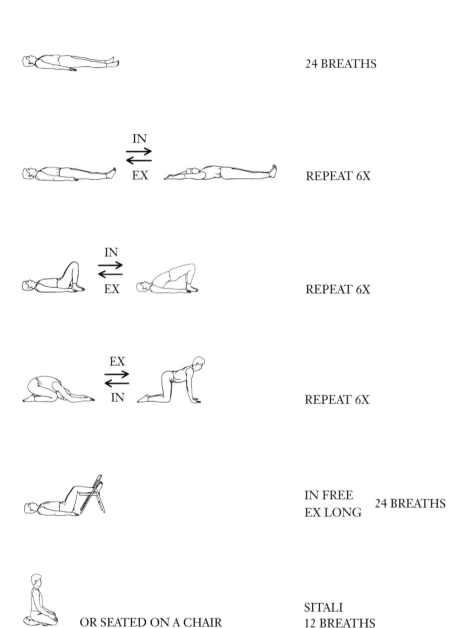

24 BREATHS

IN
EX
REPEAT 6X

IN
EX
REPEAT 6X

EX
IN
REPEAT 6X

IN FREE
EX LONG   24 BREATHS

OR SEATED ON A CHAIR

SITALI
12 BREATHS

Case 2
Finance Executive — Fourth Lesson — Evening Practice

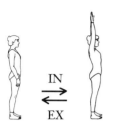

IN
EX

REPEAT 6X

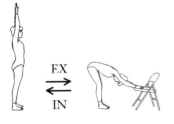

EX
IN

WAIT 4 SECONDS
AFTER EXHALE   REPEAT 6X

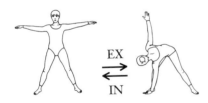

EX
IN

REPEAT 6X EACH SIDE

EX
IN

REPEAT 6X

IN
EX

REPEAT 6X

REST

IN - FREE
EX - 6   12 BREATHS
WAIT - 3

A Final Caution: The Misuses of a Yoga Practice

Any therapeutic practice of merit has the power to bring about remarkable change. Unfortunately, the very fact that these practices have power means that when used poorly, they can also bring about undesirable change. In the case of yoga, practice is too frequently done without proper knowledge or instruction, or with an ambition that can cause considerable problems for the unwary student.

Yoga is a slow, reflective process whose benefit is derived from the process itself. A well-executed practice automatically leads you to reflect on your experience. You learn to read your own body, breath, and mind. You gain the knowledge and awareness of what to do, what to give up, what to change, and when to do so, whether the practice be asana, pranayama or dhyana. Without this reflection, supported by proper technical information and guidance, the very basis of the practice is missing.

One of the most typical misuses of yoga is the practice of postures that look dramatic and impressive, such as headstand or shoulderstand, but which are entirely inappropriate for the particular student. If you are not reflective, if you have not had sufficient instruction, or if you are attached to the drama of the pose, you will not recognize when you are doing yourself harm.

A typical misuse is the inappropriate practice of a particular posture reputed to bring about a desired end. For example, a young boy who was a student came to us in basically good health, but with one complaint. He had numbness in his fingers that made him unable to hold and use a pen. Upon further examination, we found that he also practiced headstand daily — in this case, for twenty minutes — because his grandfather had told him it would help him do well on his exams. Observation again led us to conclude that the boy's body was not properly conditioned to do the pose, and we recommended that he delete headstand and follow a practice that would prepare him for the posture.

This case is not at all atypical. There are many cases of problems such as numbness in the arms, speech distortion, and so on, that result from the *inappropriate* use of headstand. Generally, the damage is the result of addiction to the pose, accompanied by a lack of reflection. As with the young boy who blindly followed his grandfather's advice, students often obey instructions that may be inappropriate to their situations or bodies. Without self-evaluation and reflection during their practice, they are unable to link the problem with its real cause.

Similar misunderstandings can apply in the practice of pranayama and meditation. A man once came to us with a cervical problem. It turned out that he had decided to follow a traditional breathing ratio that he had found in a book — a ratio of 1:4:2:1, in which he was practicing a breath retention of twenty-four seconds. He had chosen this particular ratio on the assumption that he was thereby retaining God within himself for twenty-four seconds on each round of breath, or for about thirty minutes a day.

It was clear that by forcing himself to retain his breath in this way he was causing a strain to his system. We recommended a different ratio, and the problem ceased. This was a case in which he inadvertantly created a health complication for himself by not having a teacher to observe him and his current state, and by assuming that the ratio in the book was "one-size-fits-all."

The student must also understand the real content of what he or she is doing in the practice of yoga. A woman once came to us complaining that, although she meditated three hours a day, she had no peace of mind. It turned out she was using meditation as an escape from her responsibilities in a large family. Real meditation should have brought her a sense of quiet, so that she could have looked at things from another perspective. Instead, she emerged from meditation irritated at having to re-enter her daily life. Meditation is not an escape.

Finally, we caution the student of yoga to be wary of self-instruction. Teaching yourself an asana practice from a book is unwise, not because the particular book you use is lacking in and of itself, but simply because no book can know the specifics of your situation. As we have said repeatedly throughout this book, the guidance of a capable teacher is critical.

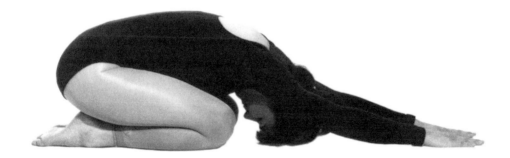

EPILOGUE

The state of personal reintegration is one in which all aspects of one's being are balanced and functioning optimally, so that reality is seen with perfect clarity. Yoga is an ideal vehicle for the movement toward this state of freedom, because its integrated approach both uses and affects every facet of human existence. In addition, it can accommodate the great diversity among people, offering a practice that can be adapted to anyone's needs and desires. In one sense, there are as many paths toward reintegration as there are people in the world; in another, more basic sense, there is only one path — the unification of oneself, the linking of the body, breath, mind and senses.

What is most important in a yoga practice is a constant sense of discovery about oneself. When a practice becomes sterile and mechanical, this cannot happen; progress comes to a halt. The key to maintaining the vitality of a practice is consistent observation by the teacher or by you, so that you can make adaptations and modifications in a timely manner.

A successful practice is one which is done regularly and is integrated with the rest of one's life. The interplay of food, activity, recreation, sleep, socializing, and so on, affect the overall quality and balance of life. The journey toward the state of yoga demands continual reassessment and redefinition of one's goals, areas of resistance, and required effort, as these various factors are in constant flux in relation to each other.

If we wish to change, to grow, and to pursue the path toward freedom, we must start from where we are right now. Movement forward must be steady, carried out with attention, reflection and gratitude. As we progress, we will notice our senses becoming disciplined and our minds less disturbed. Our attitudes toward ourselves and others will change. We will notice that we no longer suffer as we once did, and that the world is, indeed, a good place to stay, to pray, and to realize. This is the journey of total personal reintegration.

ABOUT THE AUTHOR

A.G. Mohan lives in India with his wife Indra where they have a private yoga therapy practice. They have worked with people in India, Europe, and the United States to help balance and heal body, breath, and mind.

Students with further questions can direct these either to:

The Nityananda Institute
P.O. Box 13310
Portland, OR 97213

or to:

A.G. Mohan
Plot No. 27 - Krishnakrupa
VGP Layout - Part A
Palavakkam
Madras - 600041 India

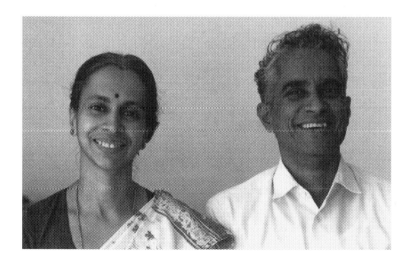

INDEX OF ASANAS

Bold indicates main description

INDEX OF TERMS

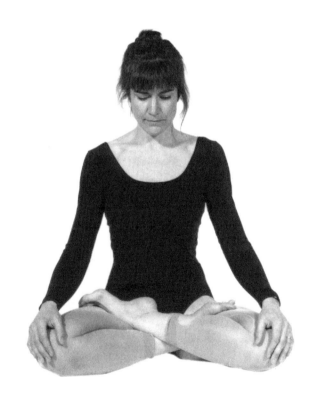

ABOUT RUDRA PRESS

We hope you enjoy *Yoga for Body, Breath, and Mind*. Rudra Press strives to publish the finest books, audios and videos on health and healing, spirituality, and hatha yoga. Practical, powerful, simple, and clear, our products are designed to meet the needs of modern life and support our customers in their quest for personal growth. Increased health, inner balance, and well-being are just a few of the many benefits contained in Rudra Press products.

Products of Related Interest

BOOKS
Yoga For Your Life/Margaret D. and Martin G. Pierce
Healing Imagery & Music/Carol A. Bush, L.C.S.W.
Secrets of Natural Healing with Food/Nancy Appleton, Ph.D.
The Breath of God/Swami Chetanananda
A Healer's Journey/Sree Chakravarti
*Stretch & Surrender: A Guide to Yoga, Health, and Relaxation for
    People in Recovery*/Annalisa Cunningham, M.A.

AUDIOS
The Balanced Body Secret/Nancy Appleton, Ph.D.
Meditation: A Guided Practice for Every Day/Swami Chetanananda

VIDEOS
Lilias! Alive with Yoga: Beginner/Lilias Folan
Lilias! Alive with Yoga: Intermediate/Lilias Folan
Lilias! Energize with Yoga/Lilias Folan
Lilias!Yoga for Better Health/Lilias Folan

**For more information on Rudra Press's complete line of products
or to request a free catalog, please call toll-free 1-800-876-7798
or fax 1-800-394-6286.**

Rudra Press
P. O. Box 13390
Portland, OR 97213